Safe Handling and Restraint of Animals

Safe Handling and Restraint of Animals

A Comprehensive Guide

Stella J. Chapman
University Centre Hartpury
Gloucestershire, UK

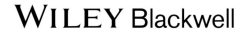

Registered Office(s)
John Wiley & Sons, Inc., 111 River Street, Hoboken, NJ 07030, USA
John Wiley & Sons Ltd, The Atrium, Southern Gate, Chichester, West Sussex, PO19 8SQ, UK

Editorial Office
9600 Garsington Road, Oxford, OX4 2DQ, UK

For details of our global editorial offices, customer services, and more information about Wiley products visit us at www.wiley.com.

Wiley also publishes its books in a variety of electronic formats and by print-on-demand. Some content that appears in standard print versions of this book may not be available in other formats.

Limit of Liability/Disclaimer of Warranty

Library of Congress Cataloging-in-Publication Data

Names: Chapman, Stella J., 1964- author.
Title: Safe handling and restraint of animals : a comprehensive guide / by
    Stella J. Chapman.
Description: Hoboken, NJ : Wiley, 2018. | Includes bibliographical references
    and index. |
Identifiers: LCCN 2017026917 (print) | LCCN 2017027887 (ebook) | ISBN
    9781119077916 (pdf) | ISBN 9781119077923 (epub) | ISBN 9781119077909 (pbk.)
Subjects: | MESH: Restraint, Physical–veterinary | Personal Protective
    Equipment–veterinary | Behavior, Animal | Animal Welfare
Classification: LCC SF760.A54 (ebook) | LCC SF760.A54 C43 2018 (print) | NLM
    SF 760.A54 | DDC 636.08/32–dc23
LC record available at https://lccn.loc.gov/2017026917

Cover Images: (First image) Courtesy of Brinsbury Campus, Chichester College;
(All other images) Courtesy of Stella Chapman
Cover Design: Wiley

Set in 10/12 pt WarnockPro-Regular by Thomson Digital, Noida, India

Printed in Singapore by C.O.S. Printers Pte Ltd

10 9 8 7 6 5 4 3 2 1

Table of Contents

Contributors

Stella J. Chapman, BVSc (Hons), MSc, ProfGCE, Grad Cert, FHEA, MRCVS
University Centre Hartpury
Gloucestershire, UK

William S.M. Justice, BVSc, MSc, MRCVS
Marwell Wildlife
Winchester, UK

Krista M. McLennan, BSc (Hons), MSc, ProfGCE, PhD
Chester University
Chester, UK

Susan M. Phillips, BVetMed, CertSAO, MRCVS
University of Surrey
Guildford, UK

Bridget Roberts, RVN, MBVNA
University of Surrey
Guildford, UK

Acknowledgement

A big thank you goes to the other contributors who share my passion for this subject and agreed to help write the book. A big thank you as well to the organizations that allowed us to use their facilities, animals and staff for the many photographs used in the book. Also thank you to my husband, Mike, whose support has been invaluable during the process of writing the book.

1

Biosecurity and Personal Equipment for Safe Handling and Restraint of Animals

Stella J. Chapman

University Centre Hartpury, Gloucestershire, UK

When handling animals it is important that your own personal safety is top priority, yet at times this can be something that is overlooked. When dealing with large animals, particularly cattle and horses, events can happen that put us at great risk and many people have been injured, or even killed, by complacency as people are in a hurry to get things done. Preparation, suitable equipment and good facilities are key to providing a safe environment, not only for yourself but also the animals that you are handling. A good knowledge and understanding of the principles of biosecurity and disease transmission are also important, in order to prevent disease spreading from animals to humans, and also from animals to animals.

1.1 Transmission of Disease

There are many ways in which disease can be transmitted and this is largely dependent on the pathogen involved. Pathogens need to be able to leave an infected host, survive in the environment, enter a susceptible person or animal and then replicate in the new host. The term *'transmission cycle'* is often used to describe this process and the cycle can either be *'direct'* or *'indirect'* (Table 1.1).

1.1.1 Zoonoses

Many pathogens are specific to humans and some specific to animals; however, there are pathogens that are capable of transmitting disease to both humans and animals. A pathogen capable of causing disease from an animal to a human is known as a zoonosis. Knowledge of these pathogens and the diseases that they cause is essential in order to prevent the transmission of disease between the animals we look after and ourselves.

Ringworm is one example of a zoonotic disease. The disease is caused by a fungus and is common in many species, including dogs, cats, horses and cattle. Many animals that are infected show no clinical signs of the disease. People will become exposed by direct contact with the infected areas on the animal and will then show clinical signs (e.g. small

Safe Handling and Restraint of Animals: A Comprehensive Guide, First Edition. Stella J. Chapman.
© 2018 John Wiley & Sons Ltd. Published 2018 by John Wiley & Sons Ltd.

Table 1.1 Transmission routes.

Direct transmission	Indirect transmission
Direct contact	Food or water
Secretions	Aerosol
Blood	Animal vectors
Urine or faeces	Fomites
Droplets	Medical devices and treatments

circular areas of reddened, inflamed skin that itch) on exposed areas (i.e. hands, neck, lower arms and face). This is prevented by careful observation of the animals that you are in direct contact with and also good personal hygiene.

There are many other examples of zoonotic diseases but it is not the intention of this chapter to provide details on these. What is important is that handlers of animals have a good basic knowledge of some of the more common zoonotic diseases that they are at risk of being exposed to when working with different species. Some of the common zoonotic diseases that handlers should be aware of are outlined in Table 1.2.

In all cases, the risk of disease transmission can be reduced by using a good handwashing technique with soap and water after handling any animal. Wearing the correct personal protective equipment (PPE) is also important.

Table 1.2 Examples of zoonotic diseases (Hiber and Darling, 2011. Reproduced with permission of John Wiley & Sons.).

Disease	Route of transmission	Prevention
Brucellosis	Direct contact; aerosol	Vaccines for sheep, cattle and goats; PPE; good hand hygiene
Campylobacter	Faeces; bodily discharges; contaminated food and water; swimming in lakes; flies can be a mechanical vector	Good hand hygiene and disinfection protocols; control of flies and rodents; prevention of faecal contamination into water and feed sources
Leptospirosis	Contaminated food, water, equipment and surfaces; spread in aerosolized urine or water; direct contact with contaminated urine	PPE; face shields should be worn if there is a risk of urine splashing; good hand hygiene; vaccines for some species, e.g. dogs and cattle
Toxoplasmosis	Ingestion of infected animal tissues or contaminated water and food; direct contact with infected faeces and soil; inhalation of aerosols	Disinfection; pregnant women should be careful when handling raw meat and avoid contact with cat faeces; wear gloves when cleaning out cat litter trays; good hand hygiene

1.1.2 Carriers

With some pathogens the host does not always show obvious clinical signs of disease. In these cases, the host acts as a *'carrier'* for the pathogen and will be capable of spreading the disease to susceptible animals.

Strangles is one example of a disease that has a 'carrier' status. The disease is caused by bacteria and is common in horses. It is important to note that with this disease there is no risk to humans becoming infected. However, strangles easily transmitted to other horses and, therefore, if you are in contact with an infected horse you must ensure that all necessary precautions are taken with regards to reducing the transmission of the disease. This will include isolation of the horse and putting biosecurity and barrier nursing protocols in place.

1.2 Infection Control

The majority of the time that people spend working with animals is with those that are healthy. However, as previously mentioned, it is not always possible to detect that the animals we are working with are ill. Therefore, it is important that handlers are aware of the methods by which the spread of disease can be prevented and controlled.

1.2.1 Biosecurity

Whereas biocontainment aims to reduce/prevent the movement of infectious diseases within a facility, biosecurity aims to reduce/prevent the introduction of new diseases into a facility from an outside source.

There are four basic principles to biosecurity:

1) selection of animals from known sources with a known health status – of particular relevance to farm animals;
2) isolation of new animals on arrival at the facility;
3) movement control within the facility;
4) sanitation using disinfection of materials and equipment and good personal hygiene.

It should be remembered that biosecurity is not just about protecting the health of the animals in your care but also about protecting your own personal health. It must also be noted that disease in animals does not always show obvious clinical signs, for example animals in the early stage of a disease or carrier animals.

1.2.2 Effective Cleaning and Disinfection

It is important when working with animals that we do so in as clean an environment as possible. Obviously, the degree to which this is done will depend to some extent on the species that we are working with and also the environment in which we are handling the animal. There are some general points to note (Dvorak and Petersen, 2009).

- *Faeces*: try to limit the amount of faecal contamination that surrounds the animal you are working with, for example always pick up faeces as soon as the dog defecates (if on a walk) or if noted in the kennels. Obviously, in a farm environment this is much harder to achieve; however, cleaning protocols should be in place and heavily soiled bedding should be removed on a regular basis.
- *Physical cleaning*: the physical removal of visible organic debris in the environment or on surfaces that you are handling an animal on is important. This may involve sweeping, brushing and scraping, depending on the organic material that you are dealing with. For example, sweeping the floor of the area where you are going to examine a horse if in a yard.
- *Sanitation*: this involves the use of hot water and some kind of detergent. These help to remove organic debris that can prevent disinfectants being effective. This has been shown to remove over 90% of bacteria from surfaces. Particular attention should be paid to floor drains and corners, as these are where debris can accumulate. A mop and bucket or bucket and washcloth with hot soapy water can be used for small areas and it is important that the water is changed several times during the process. For larger areas, mechanical washers that will remove organic debris can be used. Some of these work under high pressure to physically remove debris, whilst others produce steam to aid with removal. Care needs to be taken with high pressure machines as this method can aerosolize, and thus potentially spread pathogens. All surfaces should be rinsed with clean water, as some disinfectants will be inactivated by detergents. Personnel should also ensure that they are wearing the correct PPE when undertaking cleaning; what is worn will depend, to some extent, on the environment in which you are working.
- *Disinfection*: which disinfectant to use will very much depend on the microorganism involved, as each varies in its ability to persist in the environment as well as in its susceptibility to a particular disinfectant (Table 1.3)

When working with any kind of chemicals you will need to ensure that relevant legislation is followed. In the United Kingdom, the Control of Substances Hazardous to Health (COSHH) 2002 is the law that requires employers to control substances that are hazardous to health (HSE, 2016a). Many of the disinfectants that are available fall under COSHH guidance and it is important that risk assessments and disinfection protocols are produced. The legislation also governs that staff are provided with training and instruction on their use and that staff health is monitored.

1.3 Assessing the Risk

Whenever you are working with animals it is important to assess the risk. Risk is defined as 'a situation involving exposure to danger'. Under the Health and Safety at Work Act (1974) in the United Kingdom, an employer is responsible for ensuring that all reasonable steps are in place to provide the employee with a safe working environment. The employee also has the responsibility to ensure that all procedures that are in place are followed.

Therefore, a risk assessment needs to be carried out to ensure that all measures have been taken to prevent an incident from occurring. In order to write a risk assessment the

Table 1.3 Physical and chemical disinfection (Dvorak and Petersen, 2009. Reproduced with permission of John Wiley & Sons.).

Method	Type	Examples
Physical disinfection	Heat	May be dry heat (flame, baking) or moist heat (steam, autoclave); generally moist heat is more effective
	Desiccation (drying)	Useful for a number of pathogens; however, some, for example feline calicivirus, may be able to persist in the environment
	Ultraviolet (UV) light	Direct sunlight or UV light can inactivate some viruses, mycoplasma, fungi and bacteria, particularly airborne particles
	Radiation	Infrequently used
Chemical disinfection	Wide number of disinfectants available and the ideal disinfectant should:	No single disinfectant is available that meets all these criteria
	• have a wide antimicrobial spectrum of action; • have efficacy in the presence of organic material; • work under a number of environmental conditions	

first step is to identify the potential hazard, which is anything that could cause harm, for example approaching a horse. The risk is the chance that somebody could be harmed by the hazard, together with an indication of how serious the harm could be (HSE, 2016b). Risk can be designated as low, medium or high; the level is determined by the species or individual animal you are dealing with and the procedure you are carrying out.

1.3.1   Standard Operating Procedures

In addition to risk assessments it is good practice to have a standard operating procedure (SOP). This is a detailed list of written instructions that can be used to satisfy compliance requirements and are recommended for all procedures that pose a potential risk to the health and safety of personnel. They should also be used as the base for everyday training of staff.

1.4   Personal Hygiene

Personal hygiene is important and a high standard should be maintained at all times.

- Fingernails should be kept short (Figure 1.1) and nail polish and jewellery should not be worn.
- Long hair should be tied back above the collar (Figure 1.2).

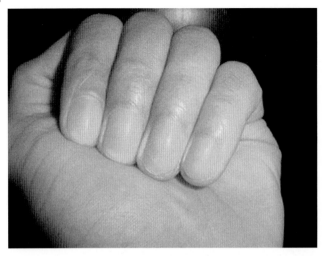

Figure 1.1 Short fingernails (Source: Courtesy of Bridget Roberts, 2016).

1.4.1 Handwashing

Hands should be washed to prevent spread of disease between animals and to humans. Hot water and soap should always be used and a good handwashing protocol such as the World Health Organisation (WHO) handwashing protocol should ideally be followed. Hands should be washed at the following times:

- before and after handling animals and leaving the facility between different animals or species;
- before and after toilet or lunch break periods;
- after glove removal and handling chemicals.

  NB: Hand gel or rub may be used, unless hands are visibly soiled.
  Gloves should be worn for the following procedures:

- handling or cleaning any bodily fluids or excreta;
- using chemicals or disinfectants.

  Ideally, a glove removal technique should be used and hands should be washed following the removal of gloves.

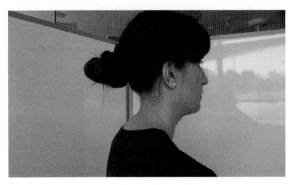

Figure 1.2 Long hair tied back above the collar (Source: Courtesy of Bridget Roberts, 2016).

1.4.2   Signs

Where possible, signs (Figure 1.3) should be placed in strategic places around animal handling facilities to remind personnel of the procedures and protocols in place. This is also very useful for new staff or visitors to the facility.

1.5   Personal Protective Equipment (PPE)

As handling an animal can be potentially hazardous to the handler, it is important to understand the risks involved, assess these risks and mitigate appropriately. One of the

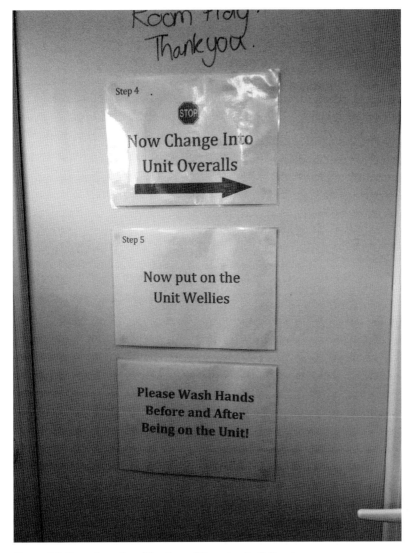

Figure 1.3 Procedure signs (Courtesy of Reaseheath College).

ways in which the handler can minimize the risk of injury or disease is by wearing the correct PPE.

It is usual for the facility where the handler is working to decide what PPE is appropriate for the species and many animal handling facilities will have a 'uniform' that they will provide to staff. It is, however, the responsibility of the person wearing the PPE to take good care of it and ensure that PPE is clean. It is good practice not to wear PPE to your home and to only wear the uniform when at work. This is not always practical or possible and, therefore, many establishments will have a uniform that can be worn at all times in clean areas, for example reception areas, and then extra PPE that is worn at specific times, such as when cleaning kennels.

All outer garments, that is overalls, should be removed prior to leaving the facility and a sticky roller should be used to remove any animal hair. The outer garments should then be placed into a bag and washed. Some facilities will provide laundry facilities; however, most people will take their PPE home to wash. It is important to ensure that the handler's own animals are not exposed to these clothes and vice versa.

1.5.1   General Points

- PPE must be worn to reduce the transfer of hair, allergens and excreta on clothing, to reduce transfer of zoonotic disease and to reduce the risk to the handler from injury.
- An animal that feels threatened is far more likely to attempt to defend itself when handled.
- Long sleeved clothing should be worn to prevent scratches on arms from sharp claws.
- Flat, enclosed toe, non-slip shoes (Figure 1.4) should be worn with companion animals and animals housed indoors to prevent trips and falls during handling or husbandry procedures.
- Stressed animals are more likely to shed potential disease agents in their faeces and other excretions. Therefore, taking steps to keep the animal as calm as possible prior to and during handling can help mitigate any risks to the handler.
- Where animals appear unwell, or are known to be carriers of disease, handlers should consider wearing gloves as extra protection, though this should not be used as a replacement for good hygiene measures and handwashing should always take place regardless after handling an animal.
- Leather gauntlets (Figure 1.5) can provide protection, but often at the expense of dexterity when handling. For large birds of prey, a leather arm guard may also be necessary.
- Steel toe-capped safety boots should be worn when handling horses and donkeys, and steel toe-capped wellington boots should be worn when working with farm animals (especially cattle).
- Eye protection is strongly recommended when handling birds with sharp pointed beaks, or other wading birds with long necks capable of reaching a handler's face.
- There are some diseases that can be transmitted to people through inhalation of small feathers or feather dust. Wearing a suitable facemask when working in aviaries, particularly those with large numbers of birds, or where ventilation is reduced, will help reduce the risk of disease transmission via this route.
- It is important when handling rodents that no perfume or scented hand cream is worn due to their sensitivity to smell.

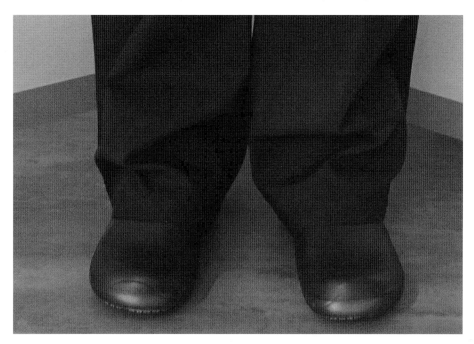

Figure 1.4 Flat, enclosed toe, non-slip shoes (Source: Courtesy of Bridget Roberts, 2016).

1.5.2 Working with Horses

In recent years, more attention has been focused on the safety of people who are working on the ground with horses. This has been in light of recent studies (BEVA, 2014; Riley *et al.*, 2015) that have looked at the risk of injury to veterinarians in the United Kingdom, and veterinary and animal science students in Australia.

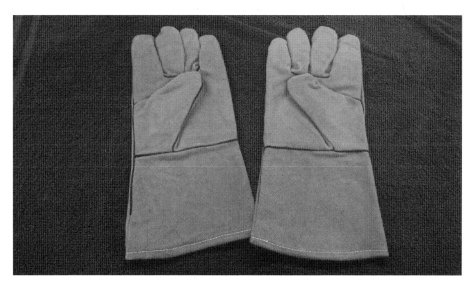

Figure 1.5 Gauntlets (Source: Courtesy of Bridget Roberts, 2016).

Veterinarians are more at risk due to the nature of their work, as they will often be carrying out procedures that are invasive, for example endoscopy of the upper respiratory tract. Also, due to the fact that veterinarians only visit horses to 'do something' to the horse, horses often will react to the presence of the veterinarian and, thus, behavioural issues (i.e. rearing) can occur. In addition, whilst veterinarians can use sedation to try to 'calm' the horse and make it easier to handle, a horse can still bite and kick whilst sedated. A large percentage of horses kept in the United Kingdom are what are known as 'pleasure' horses. They are generally owned by people who will have a varying ability in being able to handle horses, as well as knowledge of behaviour and training of horses. The study conducted by BEVA in 2014 found that a large percentage of injuries to veterinarians occurred when pleasure horses were being treated and the owner of the horse was the handler. It needs to be remembered that it is the responsibility of everyone involved with handling of the horse to ensure that safety is the main priority and to take every possible step to ensure that risk of injury is minimal. To this end, more emphasis has been placed in recent years with the use of PPE by handlers of horses on the ground, in particular with regards to the wearing of steel toe-capped boots, safety helmets and gloves.

Key Points

- When dealing with large animals, particularly cattle and horses, events can happen that put us at great risk and many people have been injured, or even killed, by complacency as people are in a hurry to get things done.
- Preparation, suitable equipment and good facilities are key to providing a safe environment, not only for yourself but also the animals that you are handling.
- A good knowledge and understanding of the principles of biosecurity and disease transmission are also important in order to prevent disease spreading from animals to humans, and also from animals to animals.
- A pathogen capable of causing disease from an animal to a human is known as a zoonosis.
- In all cases, the risk of disease transmission can be reduced by using a good handwashing technique with soap and water after handling any animal.
- Biosecurity aims to reduce/prevent the introduction of new diseases into a facility from an outside source.
- Biocontainment aims to reduce/prevent the movement of infectious diseases within a facility.
- Whenever you are working with animals it is important to assess the risk.
- One of the ways in which the handler can minimize the risk of injury or disease is by wearing the correct PPE.
- An animal that feels threatened is far more likely to attempt to defend itself when handled.

Self-assessment Questions

1   What is a zoonotic disease?
   a A disease transmitted from animal to animal.
   b A disease transmitted from humans to animals.

    c A disease transmitted from animal to humans.

    d All three of the above.

2   PPE is the abbreviation for?

    a Particular Personal Equipment.

    b Personal Protective Equipment.

    c Personal Particular Equipment.

    d Protective Personal Equipment.

3   What are the four basic principles to biosecurity?

4   What are standard operating procedures (SOPs)?

5   Why is good hand hygiene important and when should you ensure that you wash your hands?

Answers can be found in the back of the book.

References

BEVA (2014) Survey reveals high risk of injury to equine vets. *The Veterinary Record*, **175**, 263. doi: 10.1136/vr.g5714

Dvorak, G. and Petersen, C.A. (2009) Sanitation and disinfection. In: *Infectious Disease Management in Animal Shelters*, (eds L. Miller and K. Hurley), John Wiley & Sons Inc, Hoboken, NJ, pp. 49–60.

Hiber, L. and Darling, K.T. (2011) Zoonotic diseases. In: *Veterinary Infection Prevention and Control* (eds L. Caveney, B. Jones and K. Ellis), John Wiley & Sons Inc, Hoboken, NJ, pp. 63–84.

HSE (2016a) COSHH basics. http://www.hse.gov.uk/coshh/basics.htm (last accessed 18 May 2017).

HSE (2016b) Controlling the risks in the workplace. http://www.hse.gov.uk/risk/controlling-risks.htm (last accessed 18 May 2017).

Riley, C.B., Liddiard, J.R. and Thompson, K. (2015) A cross-sectional study of horse-related injuries in veterinary and animal science students at an Australian university. *Animals*, **5** (4), 951–964. doi: 10.3390/ani5040392.

Further Reading

Anon (ND) What is a Standard Operating Procedure? SOP – Standard Operating Procedure. http://www.sop-standard-operating-procedure.com/; last accessed 18 May 2017.

National Animal Disease Information Service (NADIS) www.nadis.org.uk (last accessed 18 May 2017).

World Health Organization (WHO) (2009) WHO guidelines on hand hygiene in health care. http://www.who.int/gpsc/5may/tools/9789241597906/en/; last accessed 18 May 2017.

2

Welfare Considerations for the Handling and Restraint of Animals

Stella J. Chapman

University Centre Hartpury, Gloucestershire, UK

The aim of this chapter is to provide the reader with some basic commentary and thought on welfare considerations that arise when handling and restraining animals. We handle animals on a daily basis and often with little thought given to the manner in which this is being done. Animals are restrained for a variety of reasons, some for the benefit of the animal (i.e. restraint for a health check), whilst others are for the benefit of humans (i.e. restraint for milking). At all times when we are handling animals we need to assess the need for this and how we can ensure that the welfare of the animal is our top priority.

2.1 The Human–Animal Bond: Domestication as a Consideration of Welfare

The process of domestication is a predominantly human-initiated activity in order to benefit humans, for example cattle kept for their meat, milk and hides. It is also an animal-initiated, ecologically constrained activity, for example the ability to live healthy lives and reproduce in proximity to humans, which has benefits for the animal. A lot of domestication models involved a single domestication event and then dispersion; these factors will be further explored in each species chapter. In reality, few mammalian and avian species have been truly domesticated and this is particularly the case for reptiles, birds and small mammals such as rodents. For every domesticated species, there is a progenitor species, for example the wolf was the progenitor species of the domestic dog. However, many progenitor species of domestic animals are extinct and, in some cases, the progenitor species is not easily identified, for example the extinct European Wild Horse is thought to be the most likely progenitor species for the domestic horse.

Understanding the process of domestication can help to minimize negative welfare consequences, as many behavioural and physical changes that we see in animals have been brought about by domestication. Selective breeding has further changed domesticated animals, leading to welfare consequences, for example respiratory difficulties with brachycephalic breeds of dog such as the pug. This is particularly the case for the domesticated dog, which is probably the animal most altered by domestication and through vigorous selective breeding programmes. It has also been suggested that dogs have lost intelligence during domestication or, alternatively, gained the ability to read very subtle human signals, also known as social cognition (Houpt, 2011). Thus, the process of domestication can have effects that are more than just about the physical appearance of the animal.

2.2 Welfare Considerations

There is no single accepted definition of animal welfare. However, *'The state of an animal as it attempts to cope with its environment'* (Fraser and Broom, 1990) has been widely accepted as one definition of animal welfare. This definition also portrays that there are positive and negative elements of welfare. Certainly, there are many times on interaction with owners and handlers that an animal will have to 'cope' and handling and restraint are good examples of this. The animals described within this book are all regarded by European Union legislation as being *'sentient'*. This implies that their welfare considerations should include both their physiological and behavioural needs. The term *'wellbeing'* is often used in to reflect sentience, with *'positive wellbeing'* or *'feeling good'* achieved by comfort, companionship and security (Webster, 2011).

We handle and restrain animals on a daily basis, often with little thought for the manner in which it is being done, from the dog being walked on the lead, to the horse being groomed in the stable and the cow being milked. We often, as well, expect animals to cooperate whilst they are being handled and restrained, and whilst we tend to focus on the task in hand, say walking the dog, we overlook that the animal may not always wish to cooperate with us. For example, whilst walking the dog, the dog sees a squirrel and tries to give chase – the immediate response from the handler is invariably to pull on the lead to bring the dog back to heel with a sharp verbal command. A form of what is known as negative reinforcement.

An animal will receive information from the external and internal environment, which is directed to the 'control centres' of the central nervous system in order to be processed (Webster, 2015). Much of this information is processed at a subconscious level. However, there will be times that a conscious response to a stimulus (whether positive, aversive or neutral) will require a degree of interpretation and an emotional response (i.e. sentient) can therefore ensue. As such, the handling and restraint of an animal can trigger either a positive, aversive or neutral stimuli and, as a result, behaviours to handling and restraint will be modified in the light of experience. This response will also be in light of the environment in which the animal is being handled or restrained.

2.2.1 The Five Needs/Freedoms and Reference to Animal Handling and Restraint

In order to provide for the physical and psychological needs of the animal to promote and hopefully achieve 'wellbeing', it is necessary to have a mechanism in place that provides guidance on how this can be achieved. The 'five freedoms' were some initial ideals that aimed to identify elements that defined an ideal state of wellbeing as perceived by the animals (Webster, 2015).

The five freedoms (Farm Animal Welfare Council, 1993) are:

1) freedom from thirst, hunger and malnutrition
2) freedom from discomfort

3) freedom from pain, injury and disease
4) freedom from fear and distress
5) freedom to express normal behaviour

Consideration of 'freedom from fear and distress' is paramount for owners and handlers, as the way in which we handle and restrain animals can either achieve this or, alternatively, cause, pain, injury and discomfort, and ultimately lead to fear and distress in the animal. Good handling techniques and the use of facilities designed to permit animals to move naturally with minimal disturbance and in the company of their own kind are vital if we wish to minimize stress to the animal.

Whilst the five freedoms were developed initially to address the welfare of farm animals, the five needs of the Animal Welfare Act (2006) arose in order to consider the welfare of all animals and to impose a 'duty of care' to owners and those responsible for the care of animals. The 'five freedoms' were also developed as a measure of poor welfare, whereas the 'five needs' strive to highlight what an animal needs in order to demonstrate good welfare, namely:

1) The need for a suitable environment
2) The need for a suitable diet
3) The need to be housed with or apart from other animals
4) The need to exhibit normal behaviour patterns
5) The need to be protected from pain, suffering, injury and disease

As suggested, both the 'freedoms' and 'needs' state that an animal should have the 'opportunity to display 'normal behaviour'. Scientists broadly agree that this is a function of two interacting factors: evolutionary history and environmental influences. Evolution affects an animal's physical characteristics and its behaviour through natural selection. For domestic animals, the effects of natural selection have largely been replaced by artificial selection by humans, who control access to resources such as food, shelter and mates. The behaviour of an animal is its most potent interaction with the environment and largely determines its success in survival and reproduction. 'Normal' behaviour is used to refer to behaviours that are usual, expected or 'natural' in terms of species–specific behaviour (Roberton and Matthews, 2012). However, we are still a long way off from being able to identify the range of behaviours that many of the species we handle display.

This is particularly notable with regards to birds, reptiles and small mammals. Recently, work has been done to consider the needs of what are now called 'non-traditional companion animals' (i.e. reptiles and birds). It is been identified that, with regards to these species, their welfare needs are so specialized that they could rarely, or indeed never, be met in a domestic environment (BVA, 2015). This has led to people questioning whether some species should be allowed to be kept as pets at all.

2.3 Types of Restraints and Implications for Welfare

It is beyond the scope of this chapter to look at all the different types of restraint that are available to help facilitate handling of animals. However, two examples are provided here to highlight the implications of their use with regards to welfare. It should also be noted that limited research has been done on the use of different restraints and their effect on the animal's welfare.

2.3.1   Dogs

Dogs are one of the most popular animals to be owned worldwide and exercising the dog is regarded as an essential everyday task for owners. There are many different ways in which people will provide exercise for their dog; however, the one thing that they will all have in common is that the dog will need to wear some form of restraint. In certain countries, legislation also states that dogs must be adequately restrained, for example legislation in the United Kingdom states that dogs must be restrained by a leash on public land (UK Government, 2015).

There are many different types of restraint that can be used and these will be explored in detail in the chapter on dogs. However, the type of restraint used can be detrimental to the dog's welfare. Even the simplest restraint that is commonly used by owners (leash attached to a neck collar) has been reported to cause damage to the neck and trachea (Landsberg *et al.*, 2012), particularly when dogs are prone to pulling – labradors are a breed known to be physically weak in this area. In these instances, newer restraints (i.e. halters and harnesses) have been developed that are designed to aid the handler control a strong dog or prevent injury amongst certain breeds of dog. There is, however, very little research that has looked at the different types of restraint and the implications of their use on the dog's welfare. A study by Grainger *et al.* (2016) looked at whether the type of restraint (neck collar or harness) used when walking a dog caused stress. The study found that no significant behavioural differences were found between the two different types of restraint. Nevertheless, dogs with a history of walking on a collar showed increased low ear position, which could indicate stress, but other motivators such as indicating appeasement toward their owners should also be considered. This study concluded that more long-term research is needed on the behavioural response to different types of restraints used in dogs.

2.3.2   Horses

When handling horses, safety of those that are working around the horse is paramount. The use of the nose twitch is a common restraint method that horse owners and handlers use to enable them to complete a task to a horse that is demonstrating aversive behaviours, for example clipping. At times, it is also used in order to prevent aversive behaviours or in conjunction with other methods, such as chemical restraint, to ensure the safety of those that are handling the horse, for example for certain veterinary procedures, such as stomach tubing. Whilst the use of the twitch is widely accepted as an additional means of restraint, its use is controversial as the twitch is often left in place for extended periods of time, for example during clipping, and many people who use the twitch are not trained in its use. This can mean that its use is detrimental to the horse's welfare.

Application of the twitch to the soft tissue of the horse's nose results in an increase in heart rate that is similar to a pain-inducing stimuli and the reaction of the animal to such stimuli. Endorphins are thought to be involved in the effectiveness of the twitch, as its action is blocked by naloxone and increases in plasma concentrations of immune-reactive beta-endorphin are seen following its application (Lagerweij *et al.*, 1984). There is little research that has looked at the effects of the twitch on horses. Ali *et al.* (2015) conducted a study assessing the influence of nose twitching during ear clipping in horses. The study was based on the concept that the twitch acts in a manner more like the effects of acupuncture than like divertive pain. The study concluded that nose twitches, when applied properly, could be considered a viable, humane restraint for short procedures. However, no indication was given of what is meant by a short procedure with regards to time. Frequently nose twitches are left in place for long periods of time or reapplied after a quick break in the procedure.

2.4 Stress and Implications for Handling and Restraint

Again, it is beyond the scope of this chapter to look in detail at the stress response in animals. Individual chapters have commented on recognized behaviours of individual species and the response to handling and restraint. An overview of some of the points to consider when handling and restraining animals with regards to the stress response is provided here.

Research has shown that behavioural indicators and physiological measurements, such as cortisol, glucose and lactate levels, taken after handling of animals will vary from baseline to extremely high (Grandin, 1997). Previous experience is a major factor associated with how stressful an animal will find a particular restraint or handling procedure (Brajon *et al.*, 2015).

2.4.1 Fear

Fear is defined by Webster (2015) as '*an emotional response to a perceived threat that acts as a powerful motivator to action designed, where possible, to evade that threat*'. The amygdala is the brain's fear centre. In addition, the stria terminalis in the brain is involved with separation distress and can be mediated by brain opioids (Grandin and Shivley, 2015). Thus, if species with a high flocking or herding behaviour (i.e. cattle and sheep) are separated from other animals, this isolation is often highly stressful (Diess *et al.*, 2009). Examples of a fearful response to handling and restraint can be seen in animals where a negative stimulus has been applied and the memory of the animal to that particular stimulus has thus been enhanced.

2.4.2 Novel Events

Novel events have been shown to be highly stressful (Dantzer and Mormede, 1983) and inherited breed differences in fearfulness may also affect the intensity of an animal's reaction; for example Brahman cross cattle have been reported to have higher cortisol levels after handling compared to cattle with no *Bos indicus* genetics (Zavy *et al.*, 1992). The age of the animal can also be a factor; younger animals may have a greater reaction, as older animals are affected by learning or habituation (Grandin and Shivley, 2015).

2.4.3 Previous Experience

Previous experience and genetic factors affecting temperament will determine how fearful an animal may become when being handled. For example, the squeeze chute that is used to handle cattle may be perceived as non-threatening to one animal; however, to another animal the novelty of it may trigger intense fear, as novelty is a strong stressor when an animal is suddenly confronted with it (Grandin, 1997).

Avoidance behaviour may often increase when an animal is subjected to a painful procedure whilst being restrained. This will be influenced by the severity of the procedure, the animal's previous experience and by genetic factors (Grandin and Shivley, 2015). Thus, it is important that at all times the emphasis should be that the handling experience is a positive one, as memories of negative handling and restraint can last a long time.

2.4.4 Selection for Behavioural Traits

With regards to animals such as cattle and horses, selection for animals with a calm temperament is often considered within breeding programmes, in order to reduce the risk of injury to handlers, as they are considered safer to handle. Behavioural tests are also becoming popular within shelter environments, in order to determine the animal's suitability for rehoming and, thus, increase the success rate for adoption (Marston and Bennett, 2003).

2.4.5 The Importance of Training to Improve Handling and Animal Welfare

Good handlers will be able to reduce stress during handling and restraint. Thus, the provision of training for people who are handling animals should be considered. However, whilst this is practical within a facility that provides housing for a large number of animals, this is not practical for the many owners of individual animals, such as dogs, cats, horses and rabbits. It is also important to consider the attitude of the handler towards the animals (Kauppinen *et al.*, 2012). Research has demonstrated that people with a positive attitude towards the animals they are handling can reduce the stress associated with the procedure (Waiblinger *et al.*, 2002).

Key Points

- Understanding the process of domestication can help to minimize negative welfare consequences, as many behavioural and physical changes that we see in animals have been brought about by domestication.
- The handling and restraint of an animal can trigger either a positive, aversive or neutral stimuli and, as a result, behaviours to handling and restraint will be modified in the light of experience.
- Good handling techniques and the use of facilities designed to permit animals to move naturally with minimal disturbance and in the company of their own kind, are vital if we wish to minimize stress to the animal.
- Research has shown that behavioural indicators and physiological measurements, such as cortisol, glucose and lactate levels, taken after handling of animals will vary from baseline to extremely high.
- Previous experience is a major factor associated with how stressful an animal will find a particular restraint or handling procedure.

- Avoidance behaviour may often increase when an animal is subjected to a painful procedure whilst being restrained.
- Provision of training for people who are handling animals should be considered.
- People with a positive attitude towards the animals they are handling can reduce the stress associated with the procedure.

Self-assessment Questions

1 What are the key differences between the five freedoms and five needs?

2 Give examples of species that are now referred to as non-traditional companion animals?

3 Which physiological parameters can be looked at in animals to measure the stress response to handling?

4 What is the function of the stria terminalis?

Answers can be found in the back of the book.

References

Ali, A., Gutwein, K., Hitzler, P. and Heleski, C. (2015) Assessing the influence of nose twitching during a potentially aversive husbandry procedure (ear clipping) using behavioural and physiological measures. Proceedings of the 11th International Equitation Science Conference, Vancouver, Canada. (http://equitationscience.com/previous-conferences/2015-11th-international-conference; last accessed 18 May 2017.)

Brajon, S., Laforest, J.P., Bergeron, R. *et al.* (2015) Persistency of the piglet's reactivity to the handler following a previous positive or negative experience. *Applied Animal Behaviour Science*, **162**, 9–19. doi: 10.1016.

BVA (2015) Policy statement on non-traditional companion animals, The British Veterinary Association (https://www.bva.co.uk; last accessed 18 May 2017).

Dantzer, R. and Mormede, P. (1983) Stress in farm animals: A need for re-evaluation. *Journal of Animal Science*, **57**, 6–18.

Diess, V., Temple, D., Liyour, S. *et al.* (2009) Can emotional reactivity predict stress response at slaughter in sheep? *Applied Animal Behaviour Science*, **119**, 193–202.

Farm Animal Welfare Council (1993) Second report on priorities for research and development in farm animal welfare. DEFRA Publications, London.

Fraser, D. and Broom, D.B. (1990) *Farm Animal Behaviour and Welfare*, CABI Publishing, Wallingford, UK.

Grainger, J., Wills, A.P. and Montrose, T. (2016) The behavioural effects of walking on a collar and harness in domestic dogs (*Canis familiaris*). *Journal of Veterinary Behaviour*, **14**, 60–64.

Grandin, T. (1997) Assessment of stress during handling and transport. *Journal of Animal Science*, **75**, 249–257. doi: 10.2527/1997.751249x

Grandin, T. and Shivley, C. (2015) How farm animals react and perceive stressful situations such as handling, restraint and transport. *Animals*, **5** (4), 1233–1251. doi: 10 3390/ani5040409.

Houpt, K.A. (2011) *Domestic Animal Behaviour for Veterinarians and Animal Scientists*, 5th edn, John Wiley & Sons Ltd, Chichester.

Kauppinen, T.K., Vesala, K.M. and Valros, A. (2012) Farmer attitude towards improvement of animal welfare is correlated with piglet production parameters. *Livestock Production Science*, **143**, 142–150.

Lagerweij, E., Nelis, P.C., Wiegant, V.M. and van Ree, J.M. (1984) The twitch in horses: a variant of acupuncture. *Science*, **225** (4667), 1172–1174.

Landsberg, G.M., Hunthausen, W.L. and Ackerman, L.J. (2012) *Behaviour Problems of the Dog and Cat*, 3rd edn, Saunders Elsevier, London.

Marston, L.C. and Bennett, P.C. (2003) Reforging the bond – towards successful canine adoption. *Applied Animal Behaviour Science*, **83** (3), 227–245.

Roberton, I.A. and Matthews, L. (2012) Normal behaviour of the legal animal is more than just what they do in the wild. Available at SSRN: http://ssrn.com/abstract=2050409 or http://dx.doi.org/10.2139/ssrn.2050409; last accessed 18 May 2017.

UK Government (2015) Controlling your dog in public. https://www.gov.uk/control-dog-public/overview; last accessed 18 May 2017.

Waiblinger, S., Menke, C. and Coleman, G. (2002) The relationship between attitudes, personal characteristics and behavior of stock people and subsequent behavior and production of dairy cows. *Applied Animal Behaviour Science*, **79**, 195–219.

Webster, J. (2015) *Management and Welfare of Farm Animals*, John Wiley & Sons Ltd, Chichester.

Zavy, M.T., Juniewicz, P.E., Phillips, W.A. and von Tungeln, D.L. (1992) Effect of initial restraint, weaning and transport stress on baseline and ACTH stimulated cortisol responses in beef calves of different genotypes. *American Journal of Veterinary Research*, **53** (4), 551–557.

3

Handling and Restraint of Dogs

Susan M. Phillips[1] and Stella J. Chapman[2]

[1]*University of Surrey, Guildford, UK*
[2]*University Centre Hartpury, Gloucestershire, UK*

The dog is a member of the order Carnivora, which is a diverse group of mammals that are all predatory in nature. The oldest ancestor of the dog is the miacines, which existed some 60 million years ago and eventually gave rise to the *Hesperocyon* (meaning western dog), which is thought to have existed some 36–38 million years ago. Current evidence suggests that the *Canidae* family (which includes wolves, coyotes, jackals and foxes) evolved completely in North America but did not migrate into Eurasia until much later in its history (Case, 2005). About 23 million years ago, *Hesperocyon* evolved into *Leptocyon*, which is thought to be the common ancestor of all today's canids (Wayne, 1993). The domesticated dog is classified as *Canis familiaris*.

Domestication of a species occurs when humans control the breeding and containment of large groups of animals and, as such, will affect a species over many generations; it involves the geographic, reproductive and behavioural isolation of the selected group from its wild population (Case, 2005). Dogs were the first animals to be domesticated, with DNA evidence suggesting that domestic dogs most likely diverged from wolves in different places, at different times, beginning as long as 135 000 years ago (Vila *et al.*, 1997). The ability to analyse genetic information has meant that it is now possible to more accurately classify the domestic dog. Mitochondrial DNA (mDNA) is genetic material that is passed from mothers to their young with no genetic recombination and this can be used to estimate evolutionary history (Case, 2005). Thus, whilst there are morphological and behavioural differences between wolves and dogs, mDNA demonstrates that the domestic dog is virtually identical to the other members of the *Canis* genus (i.e. wolves).

Following domestication, selective breeding in different areas of the world resulted in the wide variety of breeds that one can see in today's dog population. It is suggested that intentional selective breeding of dogs began between 3000–5000 years ago. However, most of the extreme alterations that are seen in modern purebred dogs are due to the intensive line breeding and inbreeding that has occurred within the last 150–200 years (Case, 2005). Estimates suggest that there are currently some 400 breeds of purebred dog worldwide; however, it recognized that over the history of the domestication of the dog, well over 1000 different breeds have been selected for (Case, 2005).

In 2015, a survey by the Pet Food Manufacturers Association (PFMA) reported that there are approximately 8.5 million pet dogs in the United Kingdom, with 24% of UK

Safe Handling and Restraint of Animals: A Comprehensive Guide, First Edition. Stella J. Chapman.
© 2018 John Wiley & Sons Ltd. Published 2018 by John Wiley & Sons Ltd.

households owning at least one dog (PFMA, 2015). In the United States, it is estimated that a total of 61 million dogs are owned, with 36.5% of households owning at least one dog (AVMA, 2012). Australia has one of the highest rates of pet ownership in the world and it is estimated that there are approximately 4.2 million pet dogs (RSPCA, ND). With regards to the rest of the world, much of the data on pet dog populations has come from the pet food industry and recent surveys indicate estimates for pet dogs are: six million in Canada; 43 million in Western Europe; 17 million in Eastern Europe; with statistics for South America, Asia and Africa being highly unreliable (Coren, 2012).

It can been seen from these figures that the dog features as one of man's most constant companions. This close relationship brings many associated benefits for both man and the dog. However, in recent years there has been an increased risk (especially in developed countries) of being bitten by these close companions. With this in mind it is important to be able to recognize and try to interpret canine behaviour and how the many things that we do on a daily basis to dogs in our care can have either a positive or negative impact.

3.1 Canine Behaviour

In addition to the wide variation in the way dogs look, there is also much variation when it comes to the temperament and behaviour of not only the many different breeds of dog that there are but also with regards to individual dogs. It is beyond the scope of this book to look at canine behaviour in depth with regards to all the breeds (and the many cross-breeds) of domesticated dog. Nevertheless, owing to the rising incidence of aggressive dog behaviour and the risk of being bitten that can arise due to handling and restraint of dogs, a greater emphasis has been placed on canine behaviour than has been placed in many of the other chapters.

In the United Kingdom between March 2014 and February 2015, approximately 7227 people needed medical attention after being 'bitten or struck' by a dog (a rise of 76% in the last 10 years), with children under nine years of age being most commonly affected (BBC, 2015). This despite the fact that the United Kingdom has specific legislation, namely The Dangerous Dogs Act (1991), which was updated in May 2014 to bring in stiffer penalties for dogs causing injury or death to a person. Similar figures have been reported worldwide, with numerous surveys being undertaken to look into the problem. This has also been a growing area of research for animal behaviourists.

When considering the behaviour of domesticated dogs, it is important to remember that behaviour is determined by both nature (genetics) and nurture (environment). and both of these factors can be influenced by humans.

3.1.1 Genetic Influences on Behaviour (Nature)

Behaviours can be classified into various types, such as care giving, care seeking, socializing, aggressive and hunting. In domesticating dogs, many of the behaviours shown by their ancestors have been selectively modified. For example, the hunting sequence of prey stalking, catching, killing and eating shown by wolves, has been ameliorated so that, usually, the actual killing bite is inhibited (Overall, 1997). Breeds such as the Border collie, watch, stalk and chase, a trait that has been used to work sheep, whereas scent hound breeds such as beagles have been selected for their ability to hunt prey by sense of smell. Much information about 'aggressive breeds' is based on data from bite statistics and expert opinion. Some of this information might be misleading in that factors such as popularity of breed and physical ability of the breed to inflict serious injury might skew data. However, some studies have shown significant differences in aggressive behaviours among breeds. In one study, golden retrievers and Labrador retrievers were amongst breeds demonstrating the least aggression (Duffy *et al.*, 2008), perhaps as a result of selection for their 'care giving' behaviours: their ability to retrieve food and to care for mates and young.

Probably the most common reason stated for behavioural differences in dogs will be those due to gender differences. Males are often noted to be more reactive, more playful, destructive and aggressive, whilst females tend to be more obedient, less active and more affectionate (Notari and Goodwin, 2007).

All these examples are, however, generalizations and will, in part, also be determined by the environment in which the dog is kept and human intervention, for example castrating of male dogs.

3.1.2   Environmental Influences on Behaviour (Nurture)

Husbandry factors, such as kennelling or company, and human interventions, such as castration or training, will affect behaviours at any stage in life but, as with other species, dogs have a period in their development when maturation of the nervous system facilitates their ability to respond to stimuli and when they are perhaps most readily influenced by experience.

The term 'sensitive' period has now replaced the use of 'critical' period when referring to the time when a small amount of experience (or a total lack of experience) will have an effect on later behaviour (Houpt, 2011). The timelines for dogs are outlined in Table 3.1.

Although Table 3.1 can provide general guidelines, the actual timescales may vary among breeds that are slow or fast to mature, and also amongst individuals. From a behavioural point of view, the socialization period is the most important, as it is during this time that puppies learn about their environment and about humans, with key behaviours being play (highest frequency during this time), dominance (with litter-mates), avoidance behaviour and, by eight weeks of age, fear reactions (Houpt, 2011).

Socialization of young puppies within the sensitive period is essential for normal development and experiences at this stage in life, both good and bad, may have a profound influence on behaviours throughout life.

Table 3.1 Sensitive periods (Houpt, 2011). Reproduced with permission of John Wiley & Sons.

Period	Age
Neonatal period	1–2 weeks
Transitional period	3 weeks
Socialization period	4–14 weeks
Juvenile period	14 weeks to sexual maturity

3.1.3 Canine Communication

Allied to their behaviours, dogs have a well-developed communication system and an understanding of the 'canine language' is important in any human/dog interaction, particularly when handling and restraining. A basic knowledge can help the handler to assess the demeanour of an individual dog, tailor an approach to intervention and gauge consequent reactions. An awareness of the dog's responses and the effect that further actions might have can impact significantly on the success of handling and prevent the introduction or escalation of adverse behaviours.

The special senses of the domesticated dog are specifically adapted to the environment the dog has been selected for.

Dogs have the five senses: taste, smell, hearing, sight and touch, and rely on the use of these to both give and receive information. Auditory (hearing) and olfactory (smell) senses are highly developed and, as a social species, touch is essential for communication. It is the first sense to develop in the puppy when mothers lick and nuzzle soon after birth, it is used for investigating and learning about the environment and most dogs enjoy tactile interaction. Whilst dogs have a comparatively less well developed sense of vision than humans, visual communication is used when in close proximity with another. A range of expressive body postures and gestures is adopted to convey information and there is evidence to suggest that attending to visual cues from humans is evolving (Case, 2005).

A basic knowledge of canine communication can help a handler assess the possible reactions of an individual dog. To handlers, the most obvious of these are vocal and visual communications. Tables 3.2 and 3.3 outline the meaning of various vocal sounds and visual postures, which should be considered in the context of the situation and in relation to each other when trying to interpret behaviour.

Figures 3.1 to 3.3 show images of dogs demonstrating behaviours outlined in Table 3.3.

- *Relaxed dog* – the dog is lying in sternal recumbency, the eyelids are relaxed and half closed and the tail is in a normal position (Figure 3.1)
- *Relaxed dogs* – the two dogs are both relaxed; however, they are showing different behaviours (Figure 3.2):
  - the Border collie is alert, ears forward, eyes open, jaw relaxed and mouth open with the tongue protruding;

Table 3.2 Vocalization and communication (Landsberg et al., 2012). Reproduced with permission of Elsevier.

Type of vocalization	Communication
Howling	Howling may be an ancestral means of keeping the pack together – it could be heard over a long distance. In the domesticated dog it may be a manifestation of a separation anxiety.
Whining	Whining or whimpering is often related to a 'care seeking' behaviour and may be an indication of distress.
Barking	Barking varies in frequency, volume and pitch. It has several possible connotations: it may be a threat, an alarm signal, care seeking or playful.
Growling	Growling may be used in play but is also used to warn or threaten.

Table 3.3 Body language and communication (Landsberg et al., 2012). Reproduced with permission of Elsevier.

Posture	Communication			
	Friendly relaxed	Fearful, appeasing	Defensive aggressive	Offensive aggressive
Ears	Up and forward or relaxed	Down, back	Down, back	Up/forward (will flatten on attack)
Head	Up	Down	Down	Up
Facial expression	Eyelids relaxed Jaw relaxed, mouth open, tongue protruding	Lip or nose licking Yawning	Lip or nose licking Yawning Raising the lip	Eyes open Bared teeth
Body	Standing, forward stance Lying down	Crouching Rolling Trembling Turning away Panting	Tense Puffing Hackles raised	Standing, forward stance Hackles raised
Tail	In normal relaxed position May be wagging, often with long sweeping movements	Tail between legs Slow tail wag	Tail between legs Slow tail wag	Tail high
Gaze	Pupils small	Pupils dilated Averting eye contact	Pupils dilated Darting eye contact	Pupils dilated Maintains eye contact

- the Labrador has her eyes half closed, the ears are relaxed and she is looking elsewhere but the head is up.
- *Anxious appeasing or submissive dog* – the head is down with a low body posture, avoiding eye contact, licking the nose and with the tail down (Figure 3.3)

3.1.4 Canine Aggression

Aggression serves a number of functions, some of which can be linked to an animals survival, for example aggression used in order to obtain food or to facilitate access to a sexual partner, and it is important for the handler to recognize that there are a number of categories of aggression (Table 3.4) and why these occur (Houpt, 2011).

3.2 Handling and Restraint of Dogs

As with all domestic species, handling and restraint of dogs may be necessary for a variety of reasons, including transport, husbandry, examination and treatment, and, as always,

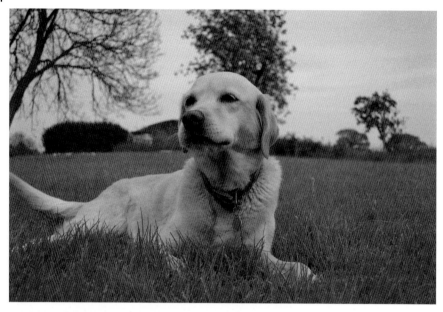

Figure 3.1 Relaxed dog (Source: Courtesy of Sue Phillips, 2015).

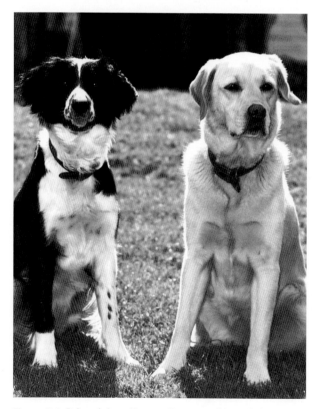

Figure 3.2 Relaxed dogs (Source: Courtesy of Sue Phillips, 2015).

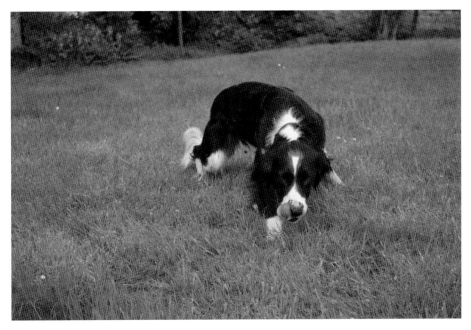

Figure 3.3 Submissive dog (Source: Courtesy of Sue Phillips, 2015).

Table 3.4 Categories of aggression (Houpt, 2011). Reproduced with permission of John Wiley & Sons.

Category	Description	Example
Social- or dominance-related	Occurs when animals live in groups; serves to establish dominance hierarchy	Dogs that normally coexist peacefully, but who fight when the owner throws a ball
Territorial	Keeps others out of a geographical area	The dog that snarls or growls at the postman – the dog is defending an area that it considers its own
Pain-induced	Develops directly out of induced pain or fear of pain	Dogs being treated at the vets and commonly seen as a defence reaction
Fear-induced	Can be related to pain, but can also be related to fear of the unknown or fear of another animal or person (with no apparent cause)	A dog retreating with the tail down and ears back
Maternal	Directly related to protection of the young	Protection of puppies by the mother following birth
Predatory	Usually directed towards another species with the main purpose being to obtain food	In dogs will be linked with the provision or non-provision of food

care must be given to the welfare of the animal during the procedure. Before beginning, various factors should be considered.

- Is the procedure necessary?
- Is the aim achievable?
- Is the animal safe?
- Is the handler safe?
- What pieces of equipment might be necessary?

Handling techniques use both psychological methods (using the animal's natural behaviours) and physical restraints (manual and chemical). Most of the problems encountered when handling dogs arise because the dog is in pain or frightened. To minimize problems:

- be patient;
- minimize stress – ensure a safe, quiet environment;
- restrict movement using a lead but use minimal restraint;
- provide distractions and rewards.

In order to achieve this:

- *Minimize stressors* – Potential environmental stressors include such things as other animals, loud noises, smells, slippery floors, ambient temperatures and so on; these should be minimized. The environment should be quiet, safe and secure, and there should be adequate space for handling.
- *Pheromones* – These are chemical substances secreted by animals to trigger various behavioural responses. Synthetic canine appeasing pheromones are now available (Adaptil: CEVA Animal Health) and diffusers may be used to generate a calming 'friendly' olfactory signal within the environment.
- *Be patient* – Allow the dog to familiarize itself with its surroundings and to strangers.
- *Be adaptable* – All dogs are individuals and no single protocol is suitable for all. Handlers should be aware of behaviours and reactions to interventions and proceed or change tactics as appropriate. Shepherd (2009) describes a ladder of aggression that depicts gestures a dog will give in response to a perceived threat. Gestures on the lower rungs include yawning, blinking and averting contact. Progression up the rungs sees the inclusion of creeping, crouched stance and lying down, and further to stiffening, growling and biting. If the dog is upset by an intervention and the intervention persists, behaviours may start to 'climb the ladder' as the dog makes increasingly clearer attempts to communicate its distress.

3.2.1 Approaching a Dog

Whether the dog is in a kennel, on a lead or free, some general principles can be applied.

- The environment should be safe and secure.
- The dog should be encouraged to approach the handler rather than the handler imposing themselves.
- Direct eye contact should be avoided.
- Threatening postures such as leaning over or cornering should be avoided. Crouching down to the dog's level may be less intimidating but care should be taken to avoid the risk of facial injury to the handler.

- Calm and simple voice commands may reassure the dog and focus its attention.
- Treats may be given as distractors and rewards but should be offered with permission of the owner. The dog may have dietary sensitivities, or the owner may prefer that treats are not given.

3.2.2   Kennelling a Dog

- *Placing in kennels* – Most dogs are probably unlikely to walk into a kennel ahead of the handler. The handler should walk in front, slowly but confidently, avoiding dragging. Once in the kennel, the dog can be turned to face the exit, the lead is gently removed and the handler leaves the kennel, walking backwards in order to keep an eye on the dog. Hand signals and voice commands such as 'sit' and 'wait' are often forgotten, but can be very useful.
- *Removing from kennels* – Removing a dog from a kennel is sometimes more challenging. A timid dog may become defensive of its 'safe haven'. The principles of approach (Section 3.2.1) apply; however, in a small kennel, it may be difficult to approach without the risk of the dog feeling cornered. If it is thought that a dog may be protective of its area, it may be beneficial to leave a collar and lead (not a slip lead) on whilst kennelled. The lead can then be reached using a grabber of some description without having to enter the kennel. Once the handler has hold of the lead and the kennel door is opened wide, the dog is often more willing to walk out.

3.2.3   Moving Around the Premises

Again, the principles of approach apply when moving a dog around the premises. Ensure the environment is safe and 'hazard free'. The path of movement should be clear, avoid confrontation with other animals and ensure restraint is secure. Double restraints should be used if possible, ideally a harness and lead plus slip lead. Alternatively, a securely fitting collar and lead, and second slip lead, may be used. If a dog has impaired mobility, additional equipment such as blankets, stretchers or trolleys (as detailed later in the chapter) may be used to aid transport.

3.2.4   Physical Restraint

Various techniques have been described for lifting and restraining dogs, but as discussed previously, no one technique suits all. Factors such as height, weight, breed, disease and temperament will all affect method, but again general principles apply.

- 'Less' is often 'more' and the minimum restraint required to be safe and successful should be used.
- Calm and friendly voice commands such as 'sit' and 'down' are often productive.
- Distractions may divert attention from the procedure and can include:
  - talking to the dog in a calm and friendly manner;
  - gently stroking, scratching or massaging;
  - a short whistle, which can often 'still' a struggling dog, thus allowing a few seconds distraction in order to perform a short procedure;
  - treats (given with the owner's consent).

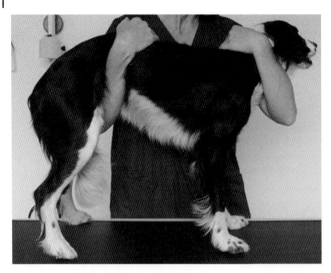

Figure 3.4 Restraint of the standing dog (Source: Courtesy of Sue Philips, 2016).

Restraint of a standing dog (Figure 3.4)
- Place one arm under the dog's neck and draw the head close to your body.
- Place your other arm under the dog's abdomen, as far back as possible to prevent the dog from sitting.
- For smaller dogs the arm may be placed over the dog and the abdomen supported by the hand.

Restraint of the sitting dog (Figures 3.5 and 3.6)
- Ask the dog to sit.
- If unsuccessful, raise the head slowly to shift the weight backwards and apply gentle pressure over the hindquarters.
- If this is resisted, with the head still raised apply gradual upward pressure behind both stifle joints.
- To maintain the sit position and restrain, place one arm under the dog's neck and cradle the head close you your body. Place your other arm over the dog's back and restrain the body snugly against you.

Restraint in sternal recumbency (Figures 3.7, 3.8 and 3.9)
- Ask the dog to lie down using an appropriate command.
- If unsuccessful, with the dog in sit restraint, stabilize the hindquarters (either with an assistant or by placing your knee behind the dog) and, with your arm over the dog's back, take hold of the forelimbs above the knee – thumb and three fingers around the legs and index finger between them.
- Lift the forelimbs, bend the elbows and gently lower the dog to sternal recumbency.
- Restrain in sternal recumbency by keeping one arm under the dog's neck, holding the head close to your body and, the other arm over the dog's back, cradling its body to yours with your forearm.

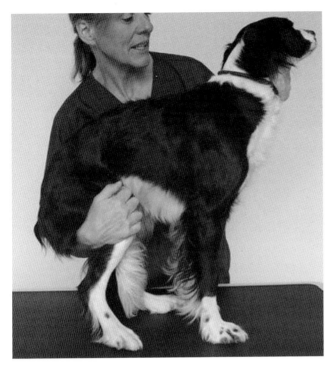

Figure 3.5 Standing to sitting (Source: Courtesy of Sue Phillips, 2016).

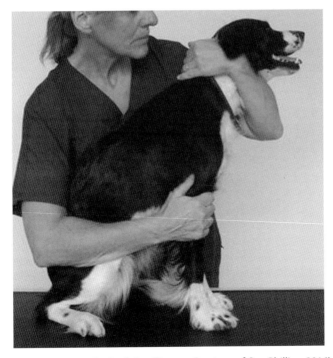

Figure 3.6 Restraint in sitting (Source: Courtesy of Sue Phillips, 2016).

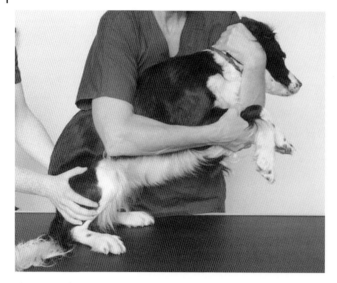

Figure 3.7 Step 1 sitting to sternal (Source: Courtesy of Sue Phillips, 2016).

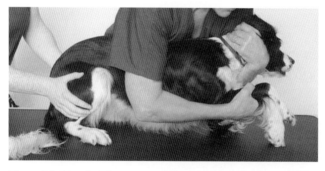

Figure 3.8 Step 2 sitting to sternal (Source: Courtesy of Sue Phillips, 2016).

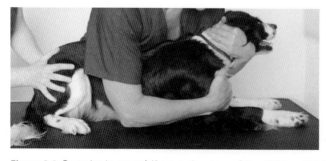

Figure 3.9 Restraint in sternal (Source: Courtesy of Sue Phillips, 2016).

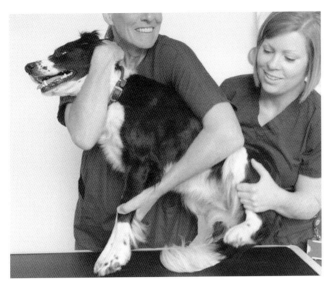

Figure 3.10 Sitting to lateral (Source: Courtesy of Sue Phillips, 2016).

Restraint in lateral recumbency (Figures 3.10 and 3.11)

From sternal recumbency

- Try rubbing the dog's abdomen, it might roll over!
- If unsuccessful, to place the dog in right lateral recumbency ask an assistant to stand on the right side of the dog and restrain, right arm under and around the neck and left arm over the dog's chest.
- Gently raise the hindquarters and rotate the pelvis to the right.
- Ask the assistant to hold the dog's forelimbs (between knee and elbow) in their left hand.
- In a coordinated fashion both handlers rotate the dog's body to the right.

From standing A dog may be placed in lateral recumbency from standing with one handler, but must be friendly or muzzled as the head is unrestrained.

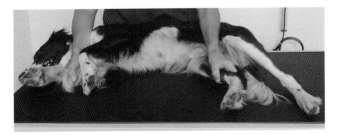

Figure 3.11 Restraint in lateral (Source: Courtesy of Sue Phillips, 2015).

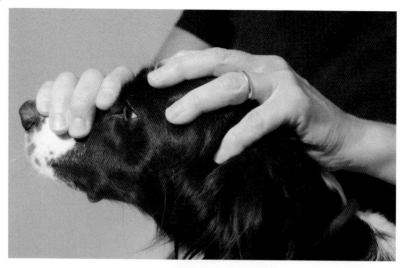

Figure 3.12 Method 1 (Source: Courtesy of Sue Phillips, 2016).

- From a kneeling position, reach over the dog and take hold of the forelimb and hindlimb closest to you, as high up as possible.
- The arm near the dog's head should be in front of the outside forelimb.
- Gently pull the limbs up, hugging the body close to you and allowing the dog to slide down your body to the ground.

To maintain lateral recumbency   Only one handler is required.

- Positioned with the dogs back against your body, place your right arm over the dog's neck, restraining the head, and hold the right forelimb between knee and elbow
- Place your left arm over the dogs back and hold the right hindlimb between the hock and stifle

Restraint of the head
There are several methods used to restrain a dog's head. The choice of method may be governed by temperament, breed and the procedure being undertaken.

- Method 1: place the right hand over the top of the head and the left hand under and around the muzzle (Figure 3.12).
- Method 2: place hands either side of the neck and head, push gently forwards (Figure 3.13).
- Method 3: roll a thick towel and gently place around the neck – this method is useful for brachycephalic breeds (Figure 3.14).

3.2.5   Lifting

Again, the method chosen for lifting a dog will depend on various factors, including the height and strength of the handler. The UK Health and Safety Executive (HSE) recommends that men can lift up to 25 kg and women 16 kg to waist height keeping

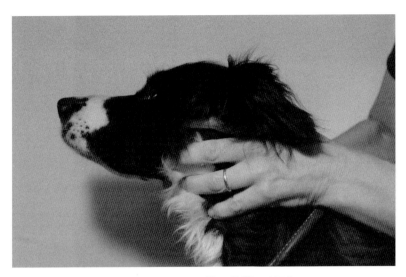

Figure 3.13 Method 2 (Source: Courtesy of Sue Phillips, 2016).

the object close to the body. There are no hard and fast rules but, generally, it is advised that two people are necessary to lift dogs weighing over 15 kg. Personnel may be able to lift heavier weights but safety could be compromised and it might not be comfortable for the dog. Larger or giant breed dogs (35 kg and over), may require three people, but it is often difficult and intimidating to fit three around the dog. In these situations it may be

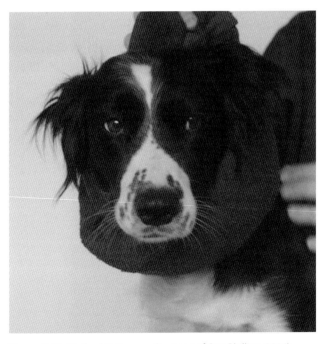

Figure 3.14 Method 3 (Source: Courtesy of Sue Phillips, 2016).

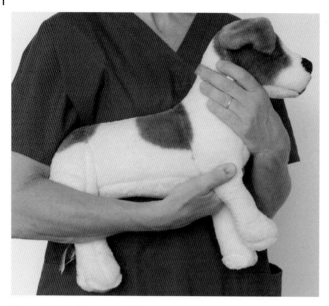

Figure 3.15 Lifting a small dog (Source: Courtesy of Sue Phillips, 2016).

more appropriate to use additional equipment such as adjustable height trolleys or stretchers.

Lifting small dogs (<10 kg)

Small dogs may be lifted in a similar fashion to cats (Figure 3.15):

- one hand or arm is used to restrain the head by placing it under and around the neck;
- place the other arm over the back and the hand under the chest to support the weight and lift, with thumb behind the outside elbow to afford some control of the leg;
- the abdomen and hind quarters can be supported by the forearm.

Lifting medium-sized dogs (10–20 kg)

Method 1 (Figures 3.16 and 3.17)

- Ensure the dog is friendly and/or ask for the head to be restrained.
- Squat down; place both arms around the dog's legs, just below the body.
- Gather and lift, keeping your back straight.

Dogs often appear comfortable with this lift but if they begin to struggle the handler has limited control and unless a muzzle or second handler is used, the head is unrestrained.

Method 2

- Place one arm under the neck, holding the head close to you to restrain.
- Place the other arm under the abdomen.

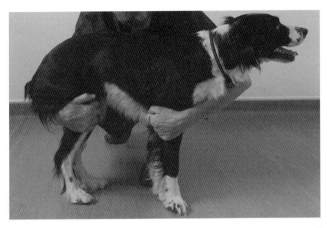

Figure 3.16 Step 1 lifting a medium-sized dog (Source: Courtesy of Sue Phillips, 2016).

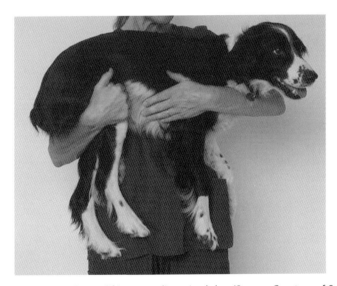

Figure 3.17 Step 1 lifting a medium-sized dog (Source: Courtesy of Sue Phillips, 2016).

The head is better restrained with this method, but both abdomen and neck will be compressed and dogs, particularly those overweight, may find the lift uncomfortable.

Method 3 Medium-sized dogs can be lifted in the same way as small dogs. The weight of the chest is well supported with this method but the hindquarters and lower back will be less contained and may be uncomfortable.

Lifting large dogs (>15 kg)
With two people (Figure 3.18):

- one person places an arm under the neck, holding the head close to restrain the head and the other arm under the chest to support weight;

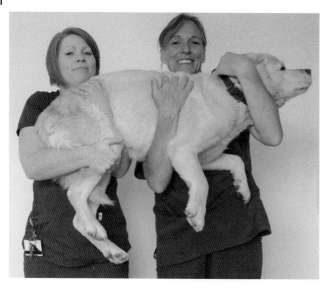

Figure 3.18 Lifting a large dog with two people (Source: Courtesy of Sue Phillips, 2016).

- the second person places one arm under the abdomen and the other arm under the hind legs and around, holding the outer stifle to secure the leg.

Lifting very large or giant breed dogs (>35 kg)
It is possible for three people to lift a large dog, one supporting the head, neck and chest, a second supporting chest and abdomen and a third standing behind to support both hind limbs. However, it may be safer for both dog and handlers if ancillary equipment is used.

3.3 Ancillary Equipment

3.3.1 Collar and Lead

Under The Control of Dogs Order (1992), UK law requires that any dog in a public place should wear a collar with the name and address of the owner either inscribed on it or on a disc attached to it. Although the order cites some exceptions, most dogs should, therefore, have a collar.

Collars should be lightweight, tight enough that dogs cannot slip out of them but loose enough to be comfortable (sufficient space for two fingers to be placed between collar and neck).

A simple collar and attached lead is often all that is required to afford adequate restraint.

3.3.2 Slip Lead

Slip leads may be used for additional security in conjunction with collar and leads or harnesses but they should be placed correctly. Slip leads are simple pieces of rope or cord

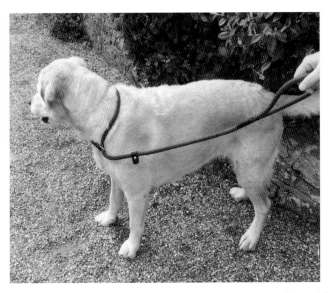

Figure 3.19 Correct fitting of a slip lead (Source: Courtesy of Sue Phillips, 2015).

that run through a metal ring to form a 'noose'. The lead may be 'slipped' to tighten or loosen the noose.

The lead should pass from the handler, over the dog's neck and around, so that the metal ring comes up from the bottom of the neck to the side of the handler. In this way the ring will run down the lead towards the handler when pressure is released, and the noose will slacken (Figures 3.19 and 3.20).

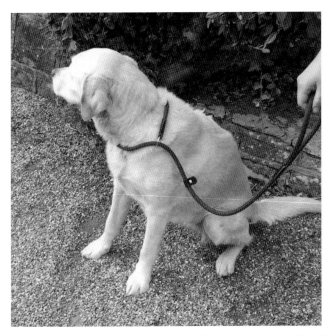

Figure 3.20 Incorrect fitting of a slip lead (Source: Courtesy of Sue Phillips, 2015).

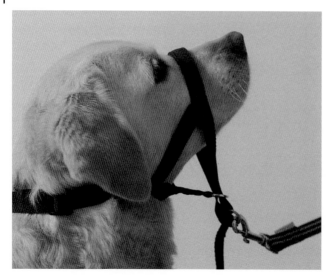

Figure 3.21 Halter restraint (Source: Courtesy of Sue Phillips, 2016).

Although some trainers advocate the use of a sharp pull to distract or deter, the UK Association of Pet Dog Trainers is strongly opposed to this.

3.3.3   Harness

Harnesses are worn around the body of the dog and, because of this, may allow the dog to pull. Used in combination with a slip lead or collar and lead, they afford comfortable restraint and are particularly useful if the dog has head or neck injuries.

3.3.4   Halters

Various restraints have been devised to discourage dogs from pulling on leads, including choke chains and pronged collars, but these train by negative experience, that is inflicting pain. Their use is extremely controversial and have been largely superseded by the introduction of halter restraints (Figure 3.21). There are various types but, as with those used for restraint of horses and livestock, they encircle the muzzle. As the dog pulls, much of the tension is directed here, with the effect of turning the dog's head without pulling unduly on the neck.

3.3.5   Muzzles

Although restraint should be kept to a minimum, there are occasions when, for the safety of personnel or other animals, it is advisable to 'muzzle' a dog. Various makes and types of muzzle are available and selection will depend on both personal preference and circumstance.

The soft fabric muzzle (Figure 3.22) is comfortable, usually well tolerated and is easy to apply, but the dog is unable to pant whilst wearing it. It should, therefore, only be used for short periods and is unsuitable for dogs with respiratory difficulties.

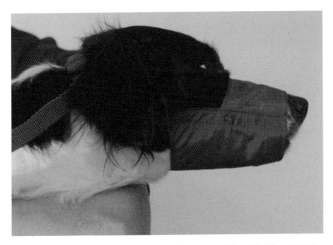

Figure 3.22 Fabric muzzle (Source: Courtesy of Sue Phillips, 2016).

The basket muzzle (Figure 3.23) is more cumbersome and dogs have been known to catch their teeth on the bars, but they allow panting, treats may be fed through the bars and they are suitable for use whilst exercising.

3.3.6 Catchers

Catch poles consist of a rigid pole with a noose (Figure 3.24). They are not commonly used but may occasionally be useful for restraining stray dogs of uncertain temperament, or aggressive dogs. Before use, it should be ensured that the noose runs smoothly and that the release mechanism is working. The noose should only be tightened sufficiently to afford secure restraint, the rigidity of the pole being used to keep the dog at a safe distance.

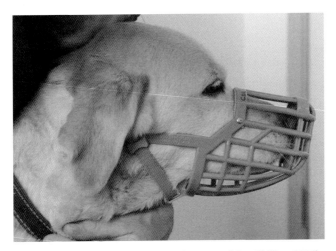

Figure 3.23 Basket muzzle (Source: Courtesy of Sue Phillips, 2016).

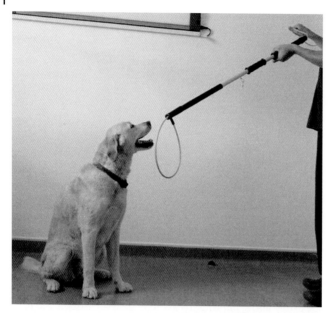

Figure 3.24 Catch pole (Source: Courtesy of Sue Phillips, 2016).

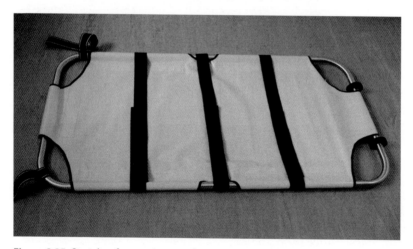

Figure 3.25 Stretcher for carrying very large or injured dogs.

3.3.7 Stretchers, Trolleys and Blankets

Very large dogs that have impaired mobility, or injured animals, may be lifted or transported with the aid of an adjustable trolley, stretcher (Figure 3.25) or large blanket. It should be ensured that sufficient personnel are available to lift comfortably and that the dog is safely secured.

3.4 Training for Restraint

As with horses, dogs often undergo a period of training, during which they learn how to do something that in the eyes of the human is either good or bad. There are several different types of learning, including habituation, instrumental learning and classical conditioning, and it is beyond the scope of this chapter to discuss them in detail. Nevertheless, an understanding of learning processes can help to create positive helpful behaviours rather than negative unwanted responses to handling and restraint.

For example, repeated exposure to a stimulus may reduce the responsiveness, a learning process known as habituation. Dogs often dislike having their feet examined. Repetitive short pleasant examinations over a period of time might reduce an adverse response.

Instrumental learning develops an association of a behaviour with a consequence. If a behaviour is desirable (sitting quietly to have feet examined), reinforcing consequences (giving a treat) will encourage this behaviour.

Classical conditioning or signal learning was first demonstrated in dogs by Pavlov where the sight of meat (unconditioned stimulus) resulted in salivation (response) and was paired with the sound of a bell (conditioned stimulus). The meat and the bell were paired repeatedly until the bell alone triggered the response of salivation. Whilst this is a positive response, this type of learning can also be responsible for a negative response, that is a dog visiting a veterinary practice for a vaccination (unconditioned stimulus) tries to bite as in pain (response) paired with the person responsible for the painful stimulus (conditional stimulus) the vet, and thus you have a negative learned response. Usually these processes are not preconceived but the handler should be aware of potential stimuli and should aim to create a positive response to a 'conditioned' stimulus.

3.5 Special Considerations

3.5.1 Handling and Restraint of Puppies

Puppies should be handled gently but securely. To lift and hold a puppy, place one hand under the chest with thumb behind an elbow, one finger between the forelimbs and remaining fingers cupping the rib cage. Support the hind quarters with the other hand. Once lifted, the abdomen and hindquarters may be supported on the forearm.

Special consideration should be given to the fact that experiences at this age, particularly during the sensitive period described previously, may significantly impact on future behavioural responses.

3.5.2 The Geriatric Dog

The older dog may have both physical and mental impairment. Commonly, 'wear and tear' on joints may affect mobility; handling techniques may have to be adapted to accommodate. Similarly, 'ageing' of the brain may reduce cognitive function.

With an ageing dog population and a rise in the number of geriatric dogs being owned, a condition similar to human senility, called cognitive dysfunctional syndrome, has been recognized (Houpt, 2011). Many older dogs are euthanized for behavioural issues, which can include house soiling and pacing and vocalizing at night, and it has been demonstrated that older dogs are also slower to learn new things.

3.5.3 Dealing with an Uncooperative or Aggressive Dog

Most dogs are uncooperative because they are fearful. Techniques for handling and restraint should follow the principles outlined previously, using the minimal restraint necessary and attempting to de-escalate rather than escalate fear. Emphasis should be placed on creating a calm, comfortable environment, use of appropriate restraint techniques and positive reinforcement of wanted behaviours.

Key Points

- Following domestication, selective breeding in different areas of the world resulted in the wide variety of breeds that one can see in today's dog population.
- The close relationship between man and dog brings many associated benefits; however, in recent years there has been an increased risk (especially in developed countries) of being bitten by these close companions.
- There is much variation when it comes to the temperament and behaviour of not only the many different breeds of dog there are but also with regards to individual dogs.
- When considering the behaviour of domesticated dogs, it is important to remember that behaviour is determined by both nature (genetics) and nurture (environment); both of these factors can be influenced by humans.
- Dogs have a well-developed communication system; an understanding of the 'canine language' is important in any human/dog interaction and, particularly, when handling and restraining dogs.
- A range of expressive body postures and gestures is adopted to convey information and there is evidence to suggest that attending to visual cues from humans is evolving.
- Aggression serves a number of functions, some of which can be linked to an animals' survival, for example aggression used in order to obtain food or to facilitate access to a sexual partner, and it is important for the handler to recognize that there are a number of categories of aggression.
- Handling techniques use both psychological methods (using the animal's natural behaviours) and physical restraints (manual and chemical).
- Most of the problems encountered when handling dogs arise because the dog is in pain or is frightened.
- Various techniques have been described for lifting and restraining dogs; however, no one technique suits all.
- The older dog may have both physical and mental impairment. Commonly, 'wear and tear' on joints may affect mobility and handling techniques may have to be adapted to accommodate. Similarly, 'ageing' of the brain may reduce cognitive function.

Self-assessment Questions

1   What is meant by the term 'critical period'?

2   Why is the socialization period for puppies so important in terms of behaviour?

3   When approaching a dog, what general principles should be applied?

4   Name five pieces of equipment that might be used in a kennel environment to control a dog that is being handled or moved?

5   State three behaviours that an anxious but submissive dog might display?

Answers can be found in the back of the book.

References

AVMA (2012) US Pet Ownership Statistics, https://www.avma.org/KB/Resources/Statistics/Pages/Market-research-statistics-US-pet-ownership.aspx (last accessed 20 May 2017).

BBC (2015) Rise in dog bite hospital admissions. http://www.bbc.co.uk/news/uk-32912084 (last accessed 20 May 2017).

Case, L.P. (2005) *The Dog: It's Behaviour, Nutrition & Health*, 2nd edn, Blackwell Publishing, Oxford, UK.

Coren, S. (2012) How many dogs are there in the world, https://www.psychologytoday.com/blog/canine-corner/201209/how-many-dogs-are-there-in-the-world (last accessed 20 May 2017).

Duffy, D.L., Hsu, Y. and Serpell, J.A. (2008) Breed differences in canine aggression. *Applied Animal Behaviour Science*, **114** (3–4), 441–460. doi: 10.1016/j.applanim.2008.04.006.

Houpt, K.A. (2011) *Domestic Animal Behaviour for Veterinarians and Animal Scientists*, 5th edn, John Wiley & Sons Ltd, Chichester.

Landsberg, G.M., Hunthausen, W.L. and Ackerman, L.J. (2012) *Behaviour Problems of the Dog and Cat*, 3rd edn, Saunders Elsevier, London.

Notari, L. and Goodwin, D. (2007) A survey of behavioural characteristics of pure-breed dogs in Italy. *Applied Animal Behaviour Science*, **103**, 118–130.

Overall, K.L. (1997) *Clinical Behavioural Medicine for Small Animals*. Mosby, St. Louis, MO.

PFMA (2015) Pet Population 2015, Pet Food Manufacturers Association (http://www.pfma.org.uk/pet-population-2015; last accessed 20 May 2017).

RSPCA (ND) How many pets are there in Australia, http://kb.rspca.org.au/How-many-pets-are-there-in-Australia_58.html (last accessed 20 May 2017).

Shepherd, K. (2009) Behavioural medicine as an integral part of veterinary practice. In: *BSAVA Manual of Canine and Feline Behaviour* (eds D.F. Horwitz and D.S. Mills), 2nd edn, BSAVA (British Small Animal Veterinary Association), Gloucester, UK, pp. 10–23.

Vila, C., Savolainen, P., Maldonado, J.E. *et al.* (1997) Multiple and ancient origins of the domestic dog. *Science*, **13** (2), 1687–1690.

Wayne, R.K. (1993) Phylogenetic relationships of canids to other carnivores. In: *Miller's Anatomy of the Dog* (ed H.E. Evans), W.B. Saunders Company, Philidelphia, PA.

Further Reading

Fowler, M.E. (2008) *Restraint and Handling of Wild and Domestic Animals*, 3rd edn, John Wiley & Sons Inc, Hoboken, NJ.

Health and Safety Executive (2012) Getting to grips with manual handling. http://www.hse.gov.uk/pubns/indg143.pdf; last accessed 6 June 2017.

Hilliard, S. (2003) Principles of animal learning. In: *Mine Detection Dogs: Training, Operations, and Odor Detection* (ed I.G. McLean), Geneva International Centre for Humanitarian Demining, Geneva.

Lane, D., Cooper, B. and Turner, L. (2008) *BSAVA Textbook of Veterinary Nursing*, 5th edn, BSAVA (British Small Animal Veterinary Association), Gloucester, UK.

Overall, K.L. (2001) Dog bites to humans – demography, epidemiology, injury and risk. *Journal of the American Veterinary Medical Association*, **218** (12), 1923–1934.

Morgan, M. and Palmer, J. (2007) Dog Bites. *British Medical Journal*, **334**, 413–417.

Sacks, J.J., Kresnow, M. and Houston, B. (1996) Dog bites: how big a problem? *Injury Prevention*, **2**: 52–54.

4

Handling and Restraint of Cats

Susan M. Phillips[1] and Stella J. Chapman[2]

[1]*University of Surrey, Guildford, UK*
[2]*University Centre Hartpury, Gloucestershire, UK*

Like the dog, the cat is a member of the order Carnivora, a diverse group of predatory mammals that share a common ancestry. The miacids, as already described in the previous chapter, split into two groups, with the miacines being the oldest ancestor for the domestic dog and the viverines being the oldest ancestor of the domestic cat. The viverines further branched into two primary lines, with evidence suggesting that the *Dinictis* was the primary cat ancestor for all cat species found today, including the domestic cat (Case, 2003). Today, the domestic cat is classified as a member of the Felidae family, a family which is divided into the subfamilies Pantherinae and Felinae. The Pantherinae group includes the tiger, lion, jaguar and leopard; the Felinae group include the lynx, puma and the genus *Felis*. The latter comprises some 26 cat species, including *Felis catus* (the domestic cat) (Case, 2003). Wildcats and domestic cats separate out into five groups, which correspond to different subspecies: the European wildcat, the Southern African wildcat, the Central Asian wildcat, Chinese desert cat and Near Eastern wildcat. These groups correspond to different subspecies and relate to geographical areas. The domesticated cat (*Felis catus*) is, however, considered taxonomically different from its progenitor species (*Felix silvestris*).

It is thought that the domestication of the cat occurred through multiple events where people tinkered with breeding or where a domestic partnership arose. Archaeological records of cat and human relationships are less abundant than dogs; the earliest consistent evidence shows that cats were most likely domesticated around 4000 BC in Egypt (Case, 2003). The most common reason for the association of cats and humans is with regards to the cat being a hunter, as evidence suggests that there was a large rodent population in Egyptian granaries and, thus, the presence of cats was tolerated by humans as they served a purpose. Unlike the dog, the cat is not completely dependent upon humans and this is demonstrated by the ability of domestic cats to return to a feral state (Case, 2003). The attitudes of humans towards cats is also different to dogs, as many people express distrust or dislike of cats.

Cats are the least genetically altered of all species and the primary physical changes that are seen are an increase in the number and variety of coat types, lengths and colours. It is only in the last 100–150 years that selective breeding has led to the development of new cat breeds with body features such as a folded ear or lack of a tail (Case, 2003).

Safe Handling and Restraint of Animals: A Comprehensive Guide, First Edition. Stella J. Chapman.
© 2018 John Wiley & Sons Ltd. Published 2018 by John Wiley & Sons Ltd.

4.1 Feline Behaviour

4.1.1 Social Structure

To handle cats safely it is important to have a basic understanding of the cat's social structure, as it enables appreciation of issues that are relevant and, thus, how the environment can be used to modify the cat's behaviour (Cory, 2010).

Whilst it has long been thought that cats are solitary by nature, recent research has demonstrated that cats can live as social animals; however, the social organization of feline groups is complicated and flexible. This allows cats to live alone or in groups of varying size, as demonstrated by feral cats who choose to live in 'colonies' or social groups whenever sufficient food resources support this structure of living (AAFP, 2004; Cory, 2010). As a solitary hunter of small prey, it is important to recognize that cats do not need the help of others, or the need to remain in groups, in order to survive and, therefore, there is little motivation to stay in a particular area or with particular individuals (Cory, 2010).

Communication varies and this reflects their social behaviour, for example queens often engage in cooperative rearing of their kittens. In addition, cats recognize individuals in their social group and have different interactions with different individuals. This behaviour is particularly important when considering integration of a new adult cat to an established group (AAFP, 2004).

Social hierarchies also exist and overt aggression (e.g. hissing, chasing, swatting) may be demonstrated when cats first establish their relationships. As long as there are no physical or environmental changes, overt aggression should cease when the relationship is established. Social relationships can change throughout life and it is important to remember that whilst the capacity to be social is inborn, specific social skills are a learned behaviour (AAFP, 2004).

4.1.2 Communication

Understanding feline communication can be quite challenging as their body language and vocalizations are more subtle than dogs (Cory, 2010). Cats, like dogs, use a variety of communication methods (Table 4.1), including visual, tactile, olfactory and auditory means.

Visual and olfactory communication are perhaps the most important in relation to the handling and restraint of cats and for this reason are worthy of more detailed discussion.

4.1.3 Visual Communication

Figure 4.1 characterizes the postures associated with various behaviours. The relaxed cat may be lying, with feet off the ground and tail loosely curled, eyes relaxed and slowly blinking (Figure 4.2). The anxious cat is beginning to prepare for flight, crouching low with all four feet on the ground (Figure 4.3). The defensively aggressive cat draws itself up and piloerects to give the appearance of being larger. Ears are flattened and tail is tucked under for protection. The offensively aggressive cat is bolder, stands tall, head and neck extended, tail straight out or extending horizontally before dropping and maintains eye contact with the source of confrontation.

Table 4.1 Communication methods (Adapted from AAFP (2004) and Cory (2010)).

Communication method	Means of communication	Reason
Visual	Body posture Tail, ear and head position Willingness to make eye contact	These are the easiest signs for people to recognize, as we rely heavily on vision
Tactile	Rubbing against others (including people) Grooming and nose touching Biting and scratching	Scent marking Used as a greeting Last defence when other signals are ignored
Auditory	Purring Trill (or chirrup), mews and meow Growling, hissing and spitting	Used primarily during contact with another individual; may indicate contentment but can be stress or pain induced Used as greeting calls Cat's sign of displeasure
Olfactory	Well-developed sense of smell Pheromones released from the face, lower back, tail and paws Odorants in urine	Smell of familiar cats can communicate friendship and acceptance Spraying can be a sign of territorial marking or insecurity

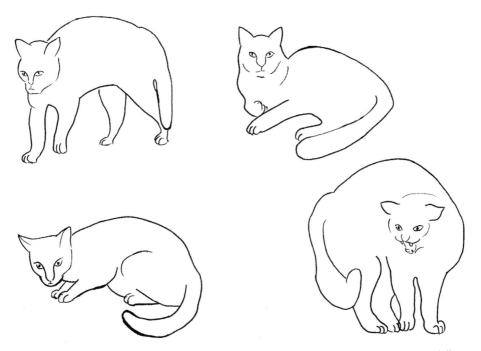

Figure 4.1 Illustration of cat behaviours as described in Table 4.2 (Source: Courtesy of Sue Phillips, 2016).

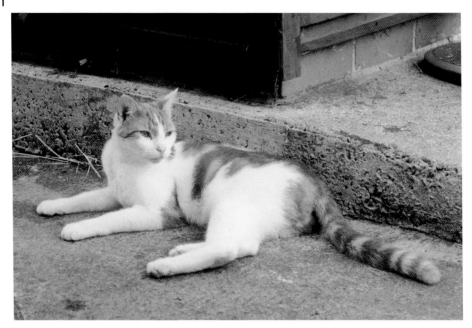

Figure 4.2 Relaxed cat. This cat is lying, feet are off the ground, eyes are half closed and facial expression is relaxed (Source: Courtesy of Sue Phillips, 2016).

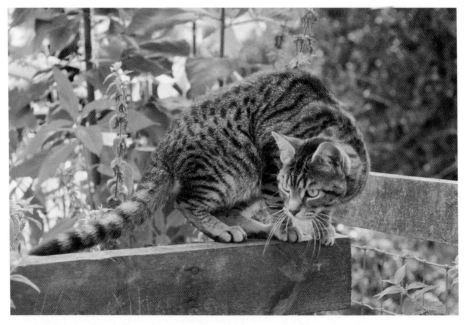

Figure 4.3 Alert, slightly defensive cat. This cat is watching the approach of a dog. Facial expression is alert but pupils are not dilated and ears are not flattened. Body posture is slightly crouched, with a degree of piloerection. All four feet are on the ground in readiness for 'fight or flight' (Source: Courtesy of Sue Phillips, 2016).

Table 4.2 The various postures and expressions associated with behaviours (Source: Overall, 1997. Reproduced with permission of Elsevier.).

Posture	Relaxed	Anxious	Defensive aggressive	Offensive aggressive
Ears	Erect when alert, relaxed when not stimulated	Ears downward, inner pinna not visible	Ears flattened downward and backward	Ears flattened but inner pinna visible
Head	Head and neck relaxed	Head and neck tucking in	Head and neck tucked in	Head up and neck extended
Facial expression	Relaxed	'Worried' expression. Whiskers backward	Mouth may be open; teeth and throat exposed	Dilated nostrils, mouth clamped
Body	Relaxed, may be standing, walking or lying – often curled up with feet off the ground	Crouching, all four feet on the ground. ready for 'flight' May tremble	Crouching or standing with hind quarters raised, and back slightly arched.	Legs straight and hindquarters elevated
Tail	Out and behind, or may be erect and curled over at tip if standing	Tail close, tucked under body	Erect bristled tail	Tail straight down or perpendicular to ground
Eyes	Pupils constricted or slightly 'off-round' Slow blink	Pupils dilated Averting gaze.	Large dilated round	Dilated oblong pupils, cat staring directly

The postures and expressions are complex and the information in Table 4.2 is much simplified. As they respond to an event, cats often send messages that lie in more than one behaviour category and their demeanour should be interpreted in the context of the situation. Facial signals change more quickly than postural ones and give the most 'up-to-date' information (Rodan, 2010).

Appearance is an obvious means of direct visual communication. Cats also send other visual messages that form an important part of their social interaction but are of less relevance to human intervention. For example, scratch marks may serve as landmarks for the cat's own use or may inform other cats, the size and height of scratches relating to the cat's physical status (Overall, 1997).

4.1.4   Olfactory Communication

The cat's sense of smell is well developed. It possesses normal olfactory cells within the nasal epithelium, with 5–10 times more olfactory epithelium than humans (Landsberg et al., 2012); it also has specialized receptors within the nasal mucosa and vomeronasal organ (VNO). The VNO is an auxiliary olfactory sense organ found in many animals. It lies close to the vomer and nasal bones in the roof of the mouth and has a direct link to the limbic system of the brain, which is responsible for emotional state. These specialized receptors detect pheromones, chemicals that are released from various glands within the body and which are capable of influencing the behaviour or physiology of other animals. Pheromones are secreted by glands situated in various parts of the body, including the face, paws and perianal areas, and are also present in urine and faeces. Cats possess facial pheromone secreting glands on their chin, lips and cheeks. Pageat and Gaultier (2003) describe five different feline facial pheromones (F1 to F5). F2 has been associated with sexual marking in tom cats. F3 is an antagonist of urine and scratch marking, appeasing the cat within its own environment. F4 is considered to be an allomarking pheromone between cats, or between cats and other species, decreasing the probability of aggressive behaviours.

Synthetic 'appeasing' pheromones (both canine and feline) have now been developed and are marketed in a variety of forms, including sprays and diffusers. Use of these chemicals in the environment may help to relieve anxiety by providing calming signals (Griffith *et al.*, 2000; Kakuma and Bradshaw, 2001).

4.1.5 Behaviour Responses

In contrast to dogs, domestic cats have retained many characteristics of their wild ancestors. They are obligate carnivores with acute hunting senses and possess heightened fight-or-flight responses (Rodan, 2010). These responses have been categorized into four groups – freeze, fiddle/fidget, flee and fight – and are perhaps better described as inhibitory, appeasement, avoidance or repulsion behaviours (Table 4.3).

4.1.6 How this can Affect Handling

An understanding of social structure and communication is important, as the interpretation of signals is very different between cats and humans. Thus, mixed messages may contribute to problems that arise when trying to handle and restrain cats, particularly if the environment or the procedure is stressful.

4.2 Handling and Restraint of Cats

The potential for compromise of the animal's welfare exists each time there is a need to handle or restrain. To minimize stress, it is important to appreciate stressors (i.e. the

Table 4.3 Behaviour responses (Source: Rodan, 2010. Reproduced with permission of Elsevier.).

Response	Behaviour
Inhibitory (freeze)	Hiding, crouching
Appeasement (fiddle/fidget)	Grooming
Avoidance (flee)	Running
Repulsion (fight)	Biting, scratching, striking

triggers of stress) and to recognize its manifestation (i.e. the signs of stress). Cats tend to hide any vulnerability and, therefore, signs of illness, pain or distress may not be easily recognized (Rodan, 2010). Their behaviour may also alter as a situation develops. Adult cats tend to be limited in their appeasement responses and usually adopt an inhibition or avoidance policy. If this is prevented, they will be pushed to repulsion (fighting) (Sundahl *et al.*, 2016) and misinterpretation of subtle messages may, therefore, result in an unnecessary escalation of problems. The use of the minimal restraint necessary to carry out a procedure safely and effectively should always be the aim, and, to this end, recognition of the feline behaviour patterns and communication signals, described previously, is important. Minimizing stressors, allowing the cats own 'coping' behaviours and recognizing emotions will all facilitate interactions between cat and handler. The recognition of emotions has been discussed but there are several ways in which the environment can be made 'cat friendly':

- Minimize stressors – Stressors include such things as loud noises, strong smells and sudden, unexpected movements:
  - provide physical separation between cats and other species (different rooms or partitions);
  - minimize waiting time;
  - keep cat carriers raised above floor level;
  - use feline appeasing pheromone diffusers;
  - keep away from loud noise;s
  - avoid the use of compounds with strong smells;
  - move slowly.
- Allow the cat's own coping behaviours – Most adult cats if frightened or challenged will adopt an inhibition or avoidance policy:
  - provide hiding places (towels or drapes over the carrier);
  - allow the cat to choose to come out of the carrier of its own accord;
  - examine the cat in its place of preference if possible;
  - avoid direct eye contact;
  - allow the cat to rub but restrict reciprocal tactile interaction to the head and neck.

4.2.1 Moving around the Premises

Cats should be moved around the premises in secure carriers and the route must be free of obstacles/stressors and so on. Top opening carriers are the easiest to use and draping with towels might help to minimize stress.

4.2.2 Removing Cats from Carriers and Cages

Before the cat is removed from any confinement, ensure that the environment is secure. Being extremely quick and mobile, even the smallest gap in a window can provide a welcome means of escape. Therefore, ensure that all windows and doors are shut. Cats are often nervous and would rather remain in their container. Ensure that the room is safe and quiet before attempting to remove them.

- Small kennels or top opening baskets:

- Initially, try to encourage the cat to come out of the container of its own free will (distractions/treats may help).
- If unsuccessful, stroke the cat's head gently, encourage exploration/rubbing and so on.
- If the cat has to be manually lifted, restrain the head and neck gently with a cupped hand, either from above or from below, and support the cat beneath the chest with the other hand. Gently lift, supporting the abdomen and hind quarters on the forearm

- Front opening baskets:
  - Try to encourage the cat to come out.
  - If unsuccessful, gently tilt or dismantle the basket (if possible).
  - Avoid dragging the cat out.
  - If necessary, move the basket to the edge of the table.
  - Hold the cat gently and ask an assistant to pull the basket slowly backwards.

Once out, place the basket **away** from the cat.

4.2.3   Placing Cats in Carriers and Cages

Anxious or frightened cats will often run or jump into the carrier seeking a place to hide. Cats that are more reluctant may need to be placed. For top opening carriers, lift and carry as described above, slowly lower into the carrier and secure the lid. Front opening carriers can be more difficult. Rather than pushing the cat in forwards, try placing them in backwards. Hold the cat with hind quarters to the carrier and slowly advance the carrier over the cat.

4.3   Physical Restraint

Cats can be a more difficult to handle than dogs. They may be more independent and less socialized, they have sharp claws, strong teeth and are very dextrous. Most of the difficulties encountered when handling cats are because they are in pain or frightened. To minimize problems:

- be patient;
- move slowly – 'slow is fast';
- minimize stress – ensure a safe, quiet environment;
- give the cat a sense of control – allow the cat to 'choose', when appropriate;
- use minimal restraint – 'less is best';
- provide distractions and rewards.

4.3.1   Lifting and Carrying Cats (Figure 4.1)

- Support the cat on one forearm, gently holding the forelegs above the carpus, thumb and three fingers around the legs and index finger between them.
- Tuck the hindlegs under your arm.
- With your other hand, either cup the head and neck from beneath, or stroke the head and neck, being ready to take a firmer hold if necessary.

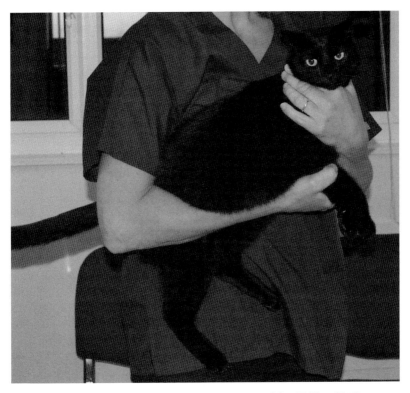

Figure 4.4 Lifting and carrying a cat (Source: Courtesy of Sue Phillips, 2016).

4.3.2   Restraint in Standing Position

- Wrap your left hand loosely around the base of the neck and shoulders.
- Stroke the top of the head and neck with the right hand, being ready to restrain further if necessary.
- The cat's body can be restrained by placing your right arm over the cat's back and confining movement of the cat's body and limbs with your forearm.

4.3.3   Restraint in Sitting Position

- Unlike dogs, cats are unlikely to sit on command.
- Place a hand around the front of the cat's chest and base of the neck, in a 'U' hold, and with the other hand, push gently above the tail, lifting the chest slightly to shift the weight backwards.
- Do not force the cat.
- Accept a standing position if the cat prefers.
- The cat can be restrained in a sitting position in similar fashion to the standing restraint (Figure 4.5).
- Keep one hand around the front of the chest and base of the neck.
- Place your other arm over the cat's back and hold the cat close to your body with your forearm.

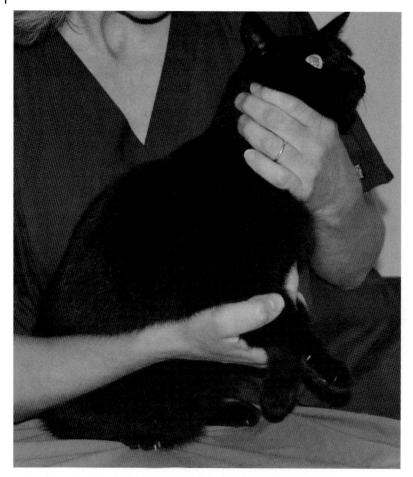

Figure 4.5 Restraint in sitting (Source: Courtesy of Sue Phillips, 2016).

- Additional control can be afforded by holding the forelimbs above the carpus, with thumb and three fingers around the legs and index finger between them.
- The hand placed in front of the chest may be moved to the back of the neck for a firmer hold, if necessary.

4.3.4 Restraint in Sternal Recumbency

- To achieve sternal recumbency from a sitting position, apply gentle pressure over the shoulders.
- Alternatively, use the same method as for the dog – from a sitting restraint, with the forelimbs held above the carpus (thumb and three fingers around the legs and index finger between them), lift the forelimbs, bend the cat's elbows and gently lower the cat to sternal recumbency.
- The cat can be restrained in sternal recumbency in the same way as for sitting restraint – maintain a hand around the front of the chest and base of neck; place your arm over the cat's back and hold the cat close to your body with your forearm (Figure 4.6); the

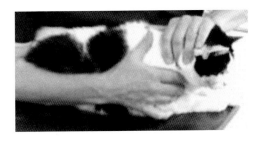

Figure 4.6 Restraint in sternal (Source: Courtesy of Sue Phillips, 2016).

hand placed in front of the chest may be moved to the back of the neck for a firmer hold if necessary.

4.3.5 Restraint in Lateral Recumbency

Many cats do not like to be restrained on their side and are not as willing as dogs to be held in this position. They can be restrained by placing on their side, dorsum to handler's body. The hind limbs are held above the hocks in one hand (first finger between the legs, thumb and remaining fingers around) and the head and neck are restrained gently with the other. A compromise can often be reached whereby the cat's front lies in sternal recumbency but the hindquarters are rotated to a lateral position.

4.3.6 Restraint for Examination of the Head (Figure 4.7)

- With the cat facing forward, hold the body to your own to prevent the cat from backing away.
- Hold the forelimbs gently, but firmly, with fingers over the cat's shoulders, preventing the cat from striking out with its claws.

4.3.7 Scruffing

'Scruffing' denotes firmly grasping the loose skin on the back of the neck. Historically it was often used as a first line of restraint but use of the method is now controversial. This 'pinch induced behavioural inhibition' (PIBI) may calm some cats, but some 'freeze' and some become distressed and more fractious when otherwise they were biddable. Nuti *et al.* (2016) researched the use of a similar restraint technique 'clipthesia'. In this procedure clips are placed along the dorsal midline of the neck. Findings suggested that clipthesia was no more stressful than scruffing but response was variable and not all cats responded positively.

In certain circumstances, to avoid injury to personnel or to perform a necessary procedure, PIBI may be appropriate but general consensus is that it should be used with consideration, not as a first line of approach and never as a means of carrying a cat without further support of its weight.

4.4 Ancillary Equipment

Many things will impact on the choice of equipment, most importantly the temperament of the cat and the experience of the handler.

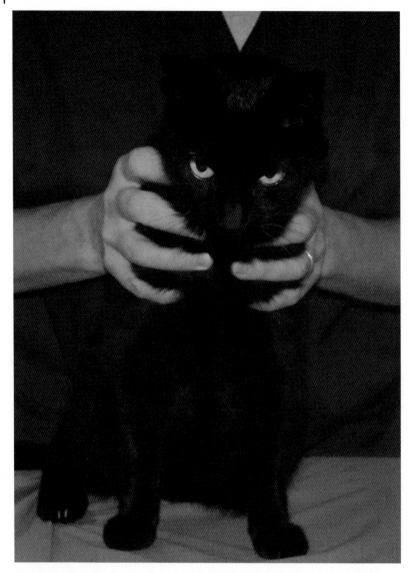

Figure 4.7 Restraint for examination of the head (Source: Courtesy of Sue Phillips, 2016).

4.4.1 Towels

Towels can be a useful adjunct to handling and restraint:

- they can provide a hiding place for the cat
- they may calm a cat by reducing visual stimuli
- they can be used to afford protection from bites and scratches

Various towel 'wraps' have been described, including the blanket wrap, the burrito wrap, the half burrito wrap, the scarf wrap and the back wrap (Yin, 2009) The type chosen depends largely on handler preference and the procedure to be undertaken. It is

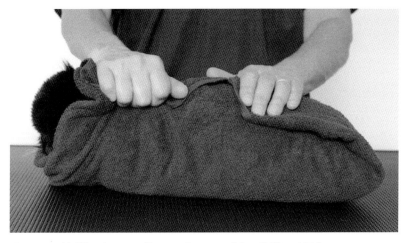

Figure 4.8 Half burrito wrap (Source: Courtesy of Sue Phillips, 2016).

beyond the scope of this chapter to describe each wrap but a few general principles apply. The towel should be sufficiently large to facilitate a secure wrap and wraps should be comfortable but snug. A method for the half burrito wrap (Figure 4.8) is (Yin, 2009):

- Lay a large towel on the table.
- Place the cat on the towel in sternal recumbency, several inches from the front edge and approximately 12 inches from one side.
- Pull the front of the towel up around the cats neck to contain the front legs.
- Take the short side of the towel over the cat and tuck under the cat snugly.
- Wrap the long side back over the cat and tuck underneath.
- Pull the back of the towel wrap up over the body to prevent the cat wriggling backwards.

4.4.2 Muzzles

Muzzles are designed to cover the eyes in order to reduce visual stimuli but will also limit the risk of bite injuries (Figure 4.9).

4.4.3 Gloves and Gauntlets

These may protect hands and arms to some extent. However, they are difficult to disinfect, may carry adverse odours and are cumbersome, as they limit the handler's dexterity.

4.4.4 Cat Bags

Various cat bags are marketed (Figure 4.10). Through the use of zips, most are designed to allow access to limbs, back and abdomen. However, getting a distressed or fractious cat into the bag is often difficult and a towel wrap may be more effective.

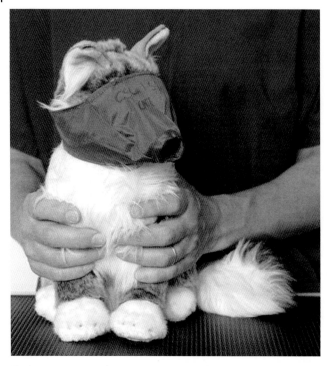

Figure 4.9 Cat muzzle (Source: Courtesy of Sue Phillips, 2016).

4.4.5 Nets

These should only be used for a quick procedure (i.e. containment of a feral cat for sedation) or in an emergency situation (i.e. capture of an escaped cat). Care must be taken that the cat does not injure toes or claws in the netting.

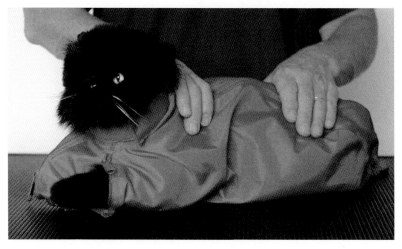

Figure 4.10 Cat bag (Source: Courtesy of Sue Phillips, 2016).

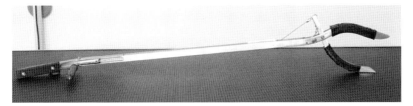

Figure 4.11 Cat grabber (Source: Courtesy of Sue Phillips, 2016).

4.4.6 Cat Grabber/Snare (Figure 4.11)

These should only be used as a last resort in emergency situations. Cats are likely to become extremely frightened by their use and aggressive behaviours will be escalated.

4.4.7 Crush Cages (Figure 4.12)

These have a moveable interior side, such that the cat can be gently confined without the need for close handling. They afford a means of superficial examination and administration of medicines, sedatives and so on. They can be useful for containing a variety of small feral or wild animal species.

4.5 Training for Restraint

Cats like familiarity (Rodan, 2010). Although perhaps not as biddable as many dogs, cats can be habituated to handling and restraint techniques such that, when they have to be employed, the cat is comfortable with the procedures and likely to be less reactive. Familiarization with carriers and restraint techniques, and positive reinforcement with

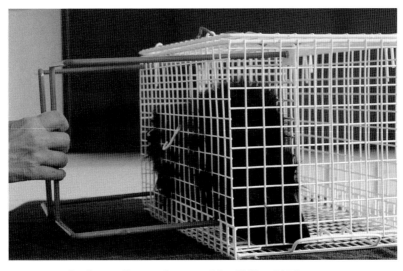

Figure 4.12 Crush cage (Source: Courtesy of Sue Phillips, 2016).

the reward of treats or toys, may help to reduce the stress of interventions. The cat is most receptive to this learning during the sensitive period described in the next section.

4.6 Special Considerations

4.6.1 Handling and Restraint of Kittens: Socialization

Socialization is the term used to describe the process of development of potentially advantageous behavioural changes as a result of exposure to novel situations involving people, other animals and new environments. Two to seven weeks of age is regarded as the feline 'sensitive' period for socialization, which is earlier than that of dogs (Turner and Bateson, 2000) and it is recommended that kittens are handled for 15 minutes per day during this time period (Houpt, 2011). This can be difficult as kittens will often remain with the breeder until after the socialization period has finished and are then secluded in their new environment and rarely introduced to unusual situations, for example restraint by strangers (Cory, 2010).

Social learning continues for many weeks with social play peaking at approximately three months of age (AAFP, 2004). Genetic variables will affect some aspects of temperament (AAFP, 2004). For example, research has shown that confident, bold fathers produce confident, bold kittens regardless of their mother's personality (McCune, 1995).

4.6.2 Behavioural Changes Associated with Ageing

It has been widely recognized that as cats age the incidence of behavioural problems increases with advancing age, and that this is often caused by underlying medical conditions. For example, hyperthyroidism, hypertension, chronic renal disease and diabetes mellitus are common conditions of older cats that are characterized by behavioural changes. As part of the normal ageing process, a decline in hearing and vision occurs, and this can lead to subsequent fear, phobias or aggression. In addition, altered sleep–wake cycles can result in wandering and increased vocalization, particularly at night (AAFP, 2004).

4.6.3 Dealing with an Aggressive of Uncooperative Cat

This is a serious problem, as it can lead to injury to other cats and people. In addition, zoonotic diseases can be spread from cats to people via scratch and bite injuries. There are a number of reasons why aggressive behaviour is displayed in cats (AAFP, 2004).

- Aggression caused by lack of socialization – Cats have a defined socialization and sensitization period and if they are not handled until 14 weeks of age, they have a tendency to be more fearful and aggressive towards people, regardless of the circumstances.
- Play aggression – Kittens often play roughly with other cats or kittens, and it is the queen and other kittens that temper this rough play behaviour. Kittens that do not learn to moderate their play behaviour will in turn play aggressively with people and,

therefore, kittens should be encouraged to play with interactive toys, rather than the feet and hands of people.

- Aggression associated with petting – As cats become socially mature, many will become less tolerant of being handled and these cats may have a form of impulse control aggression.
- Redirected aggression – Can occur when a cat is highly aroused by an outdoor cat (or other animal) and then redirects that aggression toward anyone nearby.
- Pain-associated aggression – This can take a number of different forms, for example a cat may attack an individual who causes pain or have lower tolerance because of pain.
- Inter-cat aggression – In these cases the signs of aggression are often subtle and occur in multicat households where the aggressor is able to control access to food, litter trays, resting and perching spots and attention by the owner. This behaviour is often noted when a new cat is introduced into the household, a resident cat has been absent and returns to the home (i.e. after a veterinary visit) and when there is competition for resources (i.e. litter trays and food).

Within the context of handling or restraining, in most instances aggressive behaviour is fear or pain induced. If the use of aggressive behaviour is successful at removing the stimulus, cats may learn from this experience and fearful or aggressive displays may begin to arise earlier (Moffat, 2008). Whilst the ancillary aids detailed above may help in the management of fractious cats, throughout this chapter emphasis has been placed on the need to minimize stressors and recognize emotions in order to be able to defuse adverse situations and promote positive desirable behaviours.

Key Points
<ul><li>Cats are the least genetically altered of all species and the primary physical changes that are seen are an increase in the number and variety of coat types, lengths and colours.</li><li>Whilst it has long been thought that cats are solitary by nature, recent research has demonstrated that cats can live as social animals; however, the social organization of feline groups is complicated and flexible.</li><li>Understanding feline communication can be quite challenging as their body language and vocalizations are more subtle than those of dogs.</li><li>Visual and olfactory communication are perhaps the most important in relation to the handling and restraint of cats.</li><li>Facial signals change more quickly than postural ones and give the most 'up-to-date' information.</li><li>In contrast to dogs, domestic cats have retained many characteristics of their wild ancestors.</li><li>The potential for compromise of the animal's welfare exists each time there is a need to handle or restrain.</li><li>The use of the minimal restraint necessary to carry out a procedure safely and effectively should always be the aim.</li><li>Most of the difficulties encountered when handling cats are because they are in pain or frightened.</li></ul>

- Although perhaps not as biddable as many dogs, cats can be habituated to handling and restraint techniques.
- Within the context of handling or restraining, in most instances aggressive behaviour is fear or pain induced.
- It has been widely recognized that the incidence of behavioural problems increases with advancing age, and this is often caused by underlying medical conditions.

Self-assessment Questions

1 What is meant by the term socialization and what age is regarded as the kittens 'sensitive' period for socialization?

2 State three behaviours you might see in a relaxed cat?

3 What additional items of equipment might you use to restrain a fractious or difficult cat?

4 State three things you would do before removing a cat from a cage?

5 House cats rub themselves against their owner's legs in order to:
   a Show affection?
   b Scent mark?
   c Ask for food?
   d Seek attention?

Answers can be found in the back of the book.

References

AAFP (2004) *AAFP Feline Behaviour Guidelines*, American Association of Feline Practitioners, Hillsborough, NJ.

Case, L.P. (2003) *The Cat: It's Behaviour, Nutrition and Health*, Blackwell Publishing, IA.

Cory, J. (2010) Feline ethology: understanding the cat. In: Proceedings of the Southern European Veterinary Conference (SEVC), 30 September to 3 October (www.ivis.org).

Griffith, G., Steigerwald, C.S. and Buffington, E.S. (2000) C. A. T. Effects of a synthetic facial pheromone on behaviour of cats. *Journal of the American Veterinary Medical Association*, **217** (8): 1154–1156.

Houpt, K.A. (2011) *Domestic Animal Behaviour for Veterinarians and Animal Scientists*, 5th edn, John Wiley & Sons Ltd, Chichester.

Kakuma, Y. and Bradshaw, J.W.S. (2001) Effects of feline facial pheromone analogue on stress in shelter cats. In: Proceedings of the Third International Congress on Veterinary Behavioural Medicine, Universities Federation for Animal Welfare, Wheathampstead, UK, pp. 218–220

Landsberg, G.M., Hunthausen, W.L. and Ackerman, L.J. (2012) *Behaviour Problems of the Dog and Cat*. Saunders Elsevier, London.

McCune, S. (1995) The impact of paternity and early socialisation on the development of cats' behaviour to people and novel objects. *Applied Animal Behaviour Science*, **45**, 109–124.

Moffat, K. (2008) Addressing Canine and Feline Aggression. The Veterinary Clinics of North America. *Small Animal Practice*, **38** (5), 983–1003.

Nuti, V., Cantile, C., Gazzano, A. *etc.* (2016) Pinch-induced behavioural inhibition (clipthesia) as a restraint method for cats during veterinary examinations: preliminary results on cat susceptibility and welfare. *Animal Welfare*, **25** (1), 115–123.

Overall (1997) *Clinical Behavioural Medicine for Small Animals*. Mosby, St. Louis, MO.

Pageat, P. and Gaultier, E. (2003) Current research in canine and feline pheromones. *The Veterinary Clinics of North America. Small Animal Practice*, **33**, 187–211.

Rodan, I. (2010) Understanding feline behavior and application for appropriate handling and management. *Topics in Companion Animal Medicine*, **25** (4), 178–188.

Sundahl, E., Rodan, I. and Heath, S. (2016) Providing feline-friendly consultations. In: *Feline Behavioural Health and Welfare* (eds I. Rodan and S. Heath), Elsevier, St Louis, MO, pp. 269–286.

Turner, D.C. and Bateson, P. (2000) *The Domestic Cat: the Biology of its Behaviour*, 2nd edn, Cambridge University Press, Cambridge.

Yin, S. (2009) *Low Stress Handling, Restraint and Behaviour Modification of Dogs and Cats*, Cattle Dog Publishing, Davis, CA.

Further Reading

Bradshaw, J.W.S. (2002) *The Behaviour of the Domestic Cat*, CABI Publishing, Wallingford, UK.

Cannon, M. and Forster-van Hijfte, M. (2006) *Feline Medicine – A Practical Guide for Veterinary Nurses and Technicians*, Butterworth-Heinemann, Edinburgh.

Fogle, B. (1991) *The Cat's Mind*, Pelham Books, London.

5

Handling and Restraint of Rabbits

Bridget Roberts[1] and Stella J. Chapman[2]

[1]*University of Surrey, Guildford, UK*
[2]*University Centre Hartpury, Gloucestershire, UK*

The European rabbit (*Oryctolagus cuniculus*) is a lagomorph of the family Leporidae and is the single progenitor of the domestic rabbit and is native to the Iberian Peninsula. Whilst there are many theories as to the timeline of events for domestication, historical evidence suggests that taming and selective breeding of rabbits began in AD 600 in French monasteries where monks kept rabbits for food (Carneiro *et al.*, 2011). Despite this, the rabbit is one of the most recently domesticated species (approximately within the last 1500 years).

The domestic breeds of rabbit demonstrate extensive variation in appearance, that is weight, body conformation, coat colour and so on, and also with regards to litter size, growth rate and behaviour (Carneiro *et al.*, 2011). There are over 80 breeds of rabbit, which fall into three main categories (Dallas, 2006).

- Normal – Similar to the wild rabbit; originally bred for meat, for example New Zealand and Dutch.
- Fancy – Mainly bred as show rabbits and have distinguishing features, for example Lop (ears), Netherland Dwarf and Flemish Giant.
- Rex and Satin – Bred for their velvety coats.

Because of these variations, they have historically been used for the production of meat and fur. Due to the many hereditary diseases that rabbits have in common with humans, this has also made them a valuable model for scientific research. In the United Kingdom alone, in 2014, some 14 000 laboratory procedures involved rabbits (Home Office, 2015).

In more recent years, they have become a very popular children's pet and in the United Kingdom they are the third most popular pet. According to a PFMA study in 2014–2015, there were approximately one million rabbits kept as pets in the United Kingdom (PMFA, 2015). However, according to many charity organizations, such as the RSPCA, and recent research (Schepers *et al.*, 2009) they are also one of the most poorly understood species with regards to husbandry and handling.

Safe Handling and Restraint of Animals: A Comprehensive Guide, First Edition. Stella J. Chapman.
© 2018 John Wiley & Sons Ltd. Published 2018 by John Wiley & Sons Ltd.

5.1   Behaviour of Rabbits

Domesticated rabbits still share many behaviours of their wild counterparts being a prey species, crepuscular or nocturnal and with well-defined daily patterns of activity (Wolfensohn and Lloyd, 2013). However, if they are frequently disturbed, which will inevitably happen with the way in which rabbits are kept in the pet environment, they will often become diurnal and periods of activity will be seen throughout the day and night (Jilge and Hudson, 2001). Being a species that in the wild lives in burrows, they also like to dig and the territory covered by a wild rabbit would be large. Thus, if they have the space they like to chase, jump, rear, bat at objects, gnaw and explore (Bayne, 2003). In the wild, rabbits live in social groups, which alter in size depending on the season, with both males and females demonstrating dominance hierarchies. Domestic rabbits also prefer to live in small groups. However, as the environment and the choice of cospecifics is in the control of humans, domestic rabbits needs often fall short of their wild counterparts. Rabbits are very territorial and this can present the owner of a rabbit with a behavioural issue, as the rabbit perceives that the owner is a threat to its territory (see later section on aggression). This is enforced by the fact that rabbits mainly communicate by smell and will scent mark their territory. Husbandry practices of regularly cleaning cages can have a direct impact on this and lead to stress and anxiety in rabbits.

It is important that rabbits are socialized from an early age so that they are able to cope with human interaction and also to different stimuli. As with many other 'prey' species, rabbits do not show overt signs of stress and, therefore, it is very important that handlers are familiar with an individual rabbits' range of 'normal' behaviours. Some behavioural signs that could indicate that a rabbit was stressed include:

- aggression to people or other rabbits, or when being handled;
- lethargy and lack of interest in the surroundings or food;
- hiding or trying to run away;
- appearing nervous;
- overgrooming or not grooming at all;
- stereotypical behaviours, that is biting water bottles/bars, circling, head-bobbing etc.

5.1.1   Communication

As with other species discussed in this book, rabbits use body language in order to communicate a range of emotions (Table 5.1).

5.2   Handling and Restraint of Rabbits

Rabbits are generally placid and amenable to being handled, especially if they are socialized and trained from an early age. They rarely bite; however, they can inflict painful wounds with their sharp claws.

A recent study (Oxley *et al.*, 2016) conducted a study looking at the various methods in which rabbit handling and restraint was portrayed in some 20 books (pet, veterinary and laboratory) published between 2000 and 2015. It concluded that a number of handling and restraint methods were used with regards to rabbits and that methods differed

Table 5.1 Body language and emotional states (Source: Adapted from RSPCA, ND).

Emotional state	Body position
Relaxed	Lying down with a relaxed body posture and legs tucked under the body; lying down with front paws pointing forward and rear legs extending sideways; laying down with body fully extended; jumping in the air with all four paws off the ground, twisting in mid-air before landing
Anxious	Crouched position with tense muscles, head held flat to the ground, ears wide apart and flat against the back, dilated pupils; may hide
Aggressive	Turns and moves away, flicking the back feet, ears may be flat against the back; sitting up on hind feet with ears pointed upwards and facing outwards, may be growling and display boxing behaviour; rabbit stands tense with body down, head tilted upwards, mouth open and teeth visible, pupils dilated, tail raised; back legs could be thumping the ground

depending on the context of the book. The aim of this chapter is to illustrate what the authors deem as handling that considers the welfare of the rabbit and that for specific, short, invasive procedures that are undertaken in a veterinary or laboratory setting, other methods may be used.

5.2.1 Basics

It is important when handling rabbits that you remain calm at all times; as a prey species, rabbits can be startled easily. Talking to and stroking the rabbit can help to reduce anxiety and, therefore, ensure that the rabbit is relaxed prior to handling. You should try to approach a rabbit in a confident manner, from the front and bend down to the rabbit's level, so that you are not towering above it (as a predator).

It is important that the environment is taken into account. Preferably, handling should be done in an environment that is familiar to the rabbit and also preferably with the company of another rabbit. Reduction of stimuli and stress can be aided by covering the eyes, either with a towel, or under the arm whilst lifting and carrying. Always place a rabbit on a non-slip surface, as they have fur covered feet and will slip and feel insecure if the surface is shiny.

Anatomical considerations include:

- Avoid covering the nostrils, as rabbits are obligate nasal breathers.
- The rabbit's spine must always be supported in a normal position to maintain the normal curvature of the spine at all times to prevent vertebral fractures.
- The hind limbs must always be supported and controlled, as rabbits can cause serious injury and deep wounds to the handler if they kick.
- Similarly, rabbits should be released from restraint slowly and only when all feet are on the ground, to prevent injury to the rabbit or handler by kicking.

Do not scruff or lift a rabbit by the ears.

5.2.2 Approach and Capture of a Rabbit

Approach confidently, from the front, and bend down to the to the rabbits level. Spend a moment talking and stroking to the rabbit until relaxed (Figure 5.1).

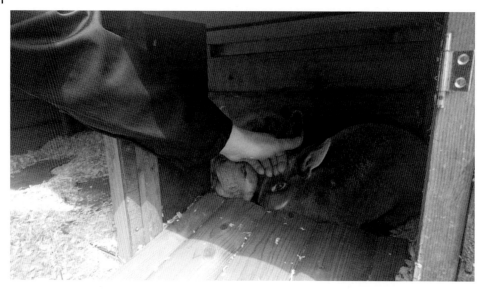

Figure 5.1 Approaching a rabbit (Source: Courtesy of Brinsbury Campus, Chichester College).

Place one hand over the shoulders and cover the eyes to calm the rabbit (Figure 5.2). Move one hand under the rabbit with the thumb and forefingers between the forelimbs, this will prevent the rabbit from running forward. Spend time gently stroking and covering the eyes to minimize stress. Once calm, you can lift the rabbit.

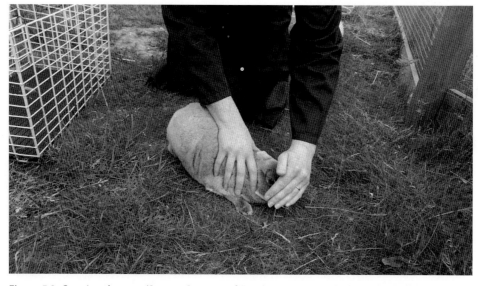

Figure 5.2 Covering the eyes (Source: Courtesy of Brinsbury Campus, Chichester College).

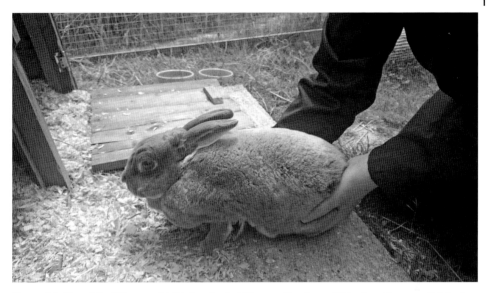

Figure 5.3 Step 1 for lifting a rabbit into a basket (Source: Courtesy of Brinsbury Campus, Chichester College).

5.2.3 Lifting a Rabbit into a Basket

Step 1 – Prepare the basket by opening the lid and placing on a flat surface. Place one hand with the thumb and fingers around the forelimbs and the other to support the hindquarters (Figure 5.3).

Step 2 – Slowly and gently rotate the rabbit so that it is laying across the forearm with the head tucked under the elbow (Figure 5.4).

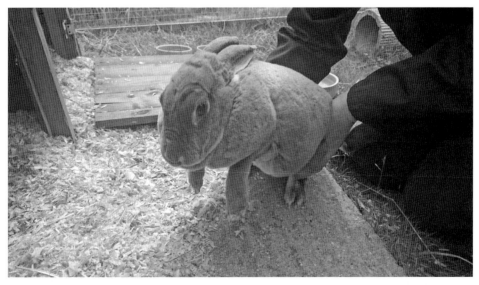

Figure 5.4 Step 2 for lifting a rabbit into a basket (Source: Courtesy of Brinsbury Campus, Chichester College).

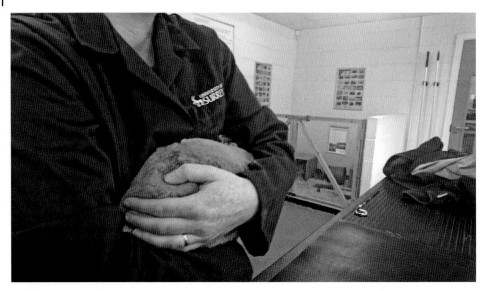

Figure 5.5 Step 3 for lifting a rabbit into a basket (Source: Courtesy of Brinsbury Campus, Chichester College).

Step 3 – Place the other arm gently on top of the rabbit, to prevent jumping (Figure 5.5).

Step 4 – The rabbit can then be carried safely and placed into the basket. Once in the basket, close the lid securely and place a towel over the basket to reduce stimulus and minimise stress (Figure 5.6).

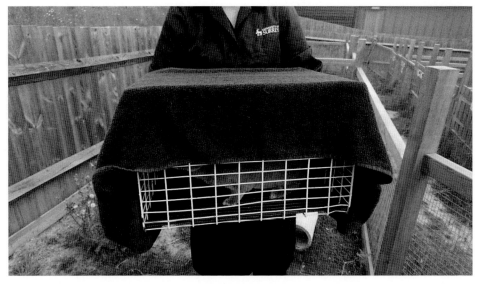

Figure 5.6 Step 4 for lifting a rabbit into a basket (Source: Courtesy of Brinsbury Campus, Chichester College).

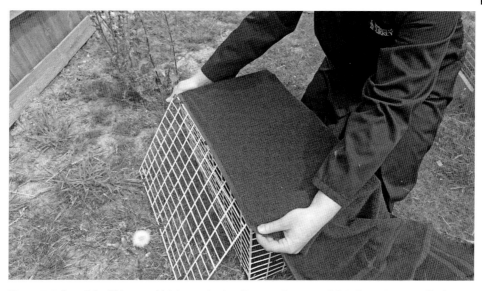

Figure 5.7 Step 5 for lifting a rabbit into a basket (Source: Courtesy of Brinsbury Campus, Chichester College).

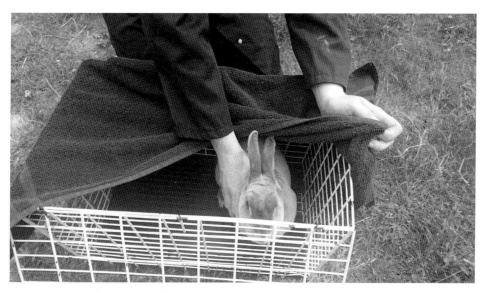

Figure 5.8 Step 5 for lifting a rabbit into a basket (Source: Courtesy of Brinsbury Campus, Chichester College).

Step 5 – When removing the rabbit from the basket, a towel may be placed under the lid to prevent jumping (Figures 5.7 and 5.8).

5.2.4 Restraint of a Rabbit on a Table

Step 1 – Place the rabbit on the table with the head tucked into the elbow and hands and arms wrapped around the body (Figure 5.9).

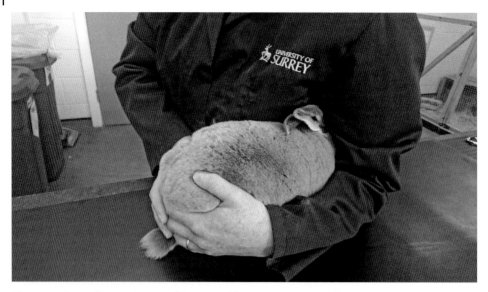

Figure 5.9 Step 1 for restraining a rabbit on a table (Source: Courtesy of Brinsbury Campus, Chichester College).

Step 2 – Place one hand over the rabbits back and the other hand over the eyes, this will prevent the rabbit from jumping or moving forward (Figure 5.10).

Step 3 – Place the rabbit on the table with the head facing away from the handler and the thumbs placed over the shoulders and index fingers in front of the forelegs, fingers wrapped around the chest (Figure 5.11).

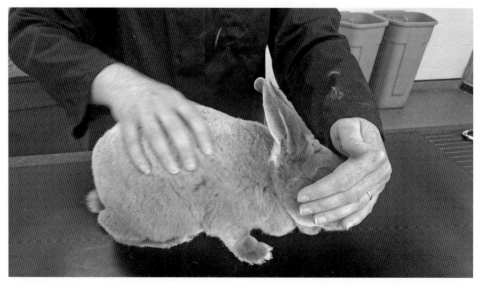

Figure 5.10 Step 2 for restraining a rabbit on a table (Source: Courtesy of Brinsbury Campus, Chichester College).

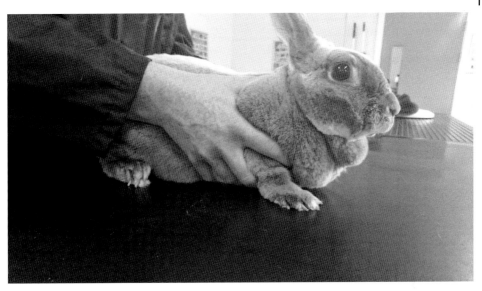

Figure 5.11 Step 3 for restraining a rabbit on a table (Source: Courtesy of Brinsbury Campus, Chichester College).

5.2.5 Restraint for Sexing or Examination of the Abdomen

Step 1 – Place one hand under the chest and grasp the forelimbs between the thumb and fingers, place the other hand around the hindquarters (Figure 5.12).

Step 2 – Gently lift and place the rabbit against your chest (Figure 5.13).

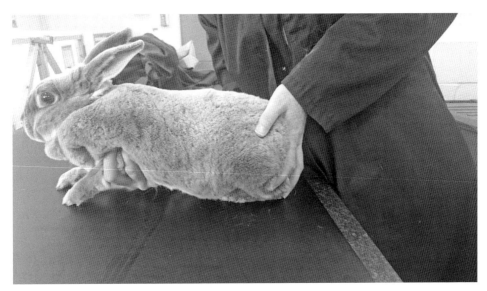

Figure 5.12 Step 1 for abdomen examination (Source: Courtesy of Brinsbury Campus, Chichester College).

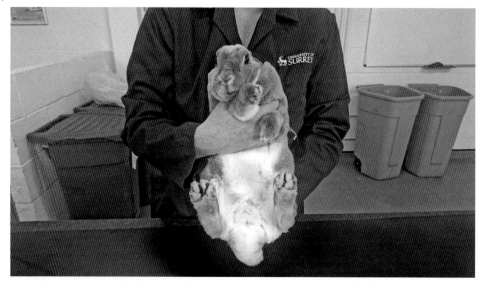

Figure 5.13 Step 2 for abdomen examination (Source: Courtesy of Brinsbury Campus, Chichester College).

5.2.6 Restraint for Aggressive Rabbits

It can be useful to use a towel (Figure 5.14) to throw over a very aggressive rabbit in order to prevent biting and scratching. The rabbit may then be scooped up in the towel safely. The towel covers the eyes, which also helps to calm the rabbit.

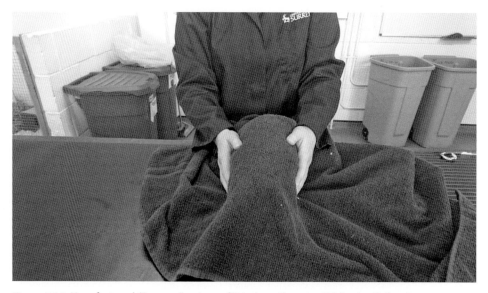

Figure 5.14 Use of a towel (Source: Courtesy of Brinsbury Campus, Chichester College).

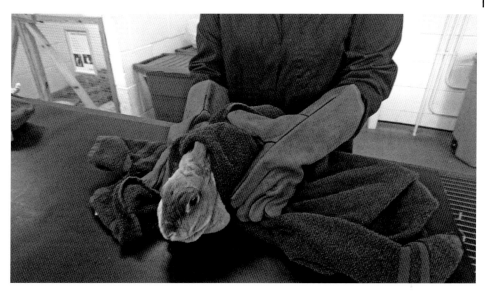

Figure 5.15 Use of gauntlets (Source: Courtesy of Brinsbury Campus, Chichester College).

Long gauntlets (Figure 5.15) may be required for handling of exceptionally aggressive rabbits (i.e. rabbits that are growling, biting or boxing). However, these will limit the dexterity of the handler.

5.2.7 Alternative Restraint Methods for Rabbits

Cat bag (Figures 5.16 and 5.17) – The rabbit may be placed in the bag to prevent scratching, as all limbs are restrained in the bag, leaving the head exposed. The two zips, either side of the forelimbs, may be unzipped to allow access to one or both limbs. This is particularly useful for intravenous catheter placement or claw clipping.

5.2.8 Towel Wrap or 'Bunny Burrito'

This is a useful restraint for stressed or fractious rabbits. It allows for examination of the head and mouth, and also for more invasive veterinary procedures, such as inserting an intravenous catheter into the marginal ear vein. Also, one foreleg can be exposed from the towel for examination and so on.

Step 1 – Lay out a large towel on a solid/non-slip table. With the handler standing behind the rabbit, place the rabbit in the middle of the towel, facing away from the handler, with the forelegs approximately 2–3 inches from the front edge of the towel (Figure 5.18).

Step 2 – Whilst keeping one hand over the rabbit's shoulders to prevent escape, fold the back edge of the towel over the lumbar region (Figure 5.19).

Step 3 – Whilst keeping one hand over the rabbit's shoulders, fold one side of the towel over the dorsum, enclosing the foreleg and ensuring that the mouth is not covered (Figure 5.20).

Step 4 – Repeat step 3 on the opposite side, then finally tuck the last towel edge under the rabbit to secure the wrap (Figure 5.21).

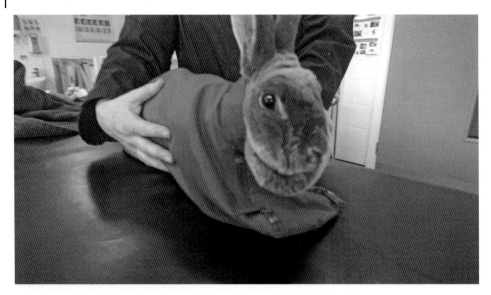

Figure 5.16 Cat bag (Source: Courtesy of Brinsbury Campus, Chichester College).

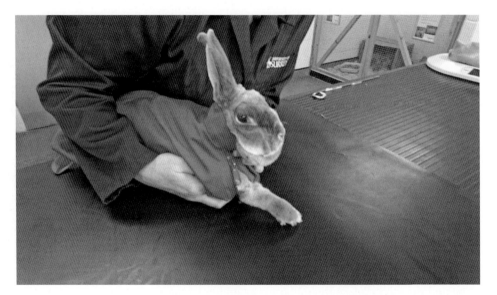

Figure 5.17 Cat bag (Source: Courtesy of Brinsbury Campus, Chichester College).

5.2.9 Tonic Immobilization

'Trancing' is sometimes advocated as a method of restraint for relaxation in rabbits. This is a fear response that causes stress and is rarely necessary in rabbit handling (McBride *et al.*, 2006). It can be achieved by placing a rabbit in dorsal recumbency and stroking the head. This will cause the rabbit to freeze and become unresponsive to stimuli. It should never be used to perform painful procedures but can be used as a last resort in aggressive or fearful rabbits.

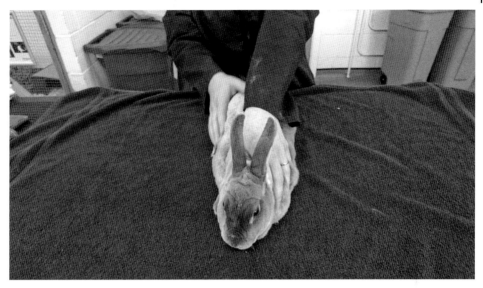

Figure 5.18 Step 1 for the Towel Wrap or 'Bunny Burrito' (Source: Courtesy of Brinsbury Campus, Chichester College).

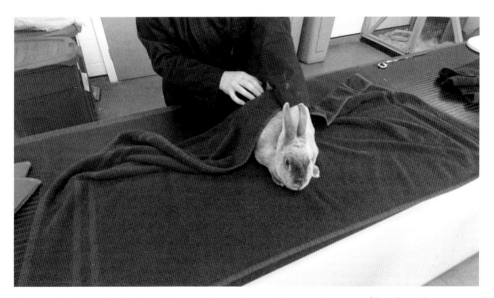

Figure 5.19 Step 2 for the Towel Wrap or 'Bunny Burrito' (Source: Courtesy of Brinsbury Campus, Chichester College).

5.3 Aggression

Rabbit aggression is fairly common and rabbits will often display this behaviour in many ways, for example biting, boxing with the front legs, growling, screaming, thumping, lunging and spraying. Handlers should take particular care when handling aggressive rabbits as they can inflict very serious injuries, particularly deep scratches or bites.

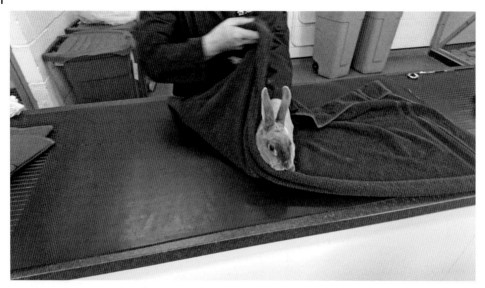

Figure 5.20 Step 3 for the Towel Wrap or 'Bunny Burrito' (Source: Courtesy of Brinsbury Campus, Chichester College).

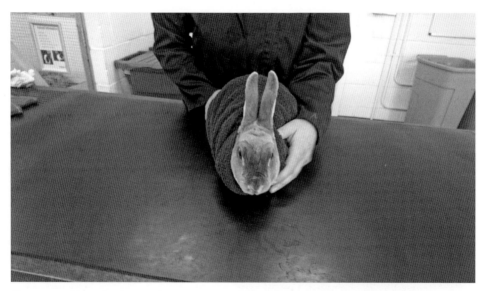

Figure 5.21 Step 4 for the Towel Wrap or 'Bunny Burrito' (Source: Courtesy of Brinsbury Campus, Chichester College).

5.3.1 Aggression as a Normal Behaviour

In the wild rabbits are a prey animal and, as such, if they feel under threat from a predator will either freeze, run away or fight. As the rabbit has eyes on the side of the head (all round vision) and large ears for detection of sound, the normal reaction to a predator would be to run away. However, if caught, the rabbit will use its teeth, claws and powerful back legs to fight.

Wild rabbits are also territorial and, as such, will defend an area against a rival group. Female rabbits will also protect nest sites and can be very aggressive in the later stages of pregnancy or when they have young in the nest.

5.3.2 Aggression as an Abnormal Behaviour

There are a number of reasons why rabbits that are kept as pets may demonstrate aggressive behaviour, including (RWAF, ND):

- Handling – Rabbits that were not handled from a young age can view the owner as a potential threat when they try to handle the rabbit or even just stroke the rabbit. The rabbit will initially freeze or try to run away; however, if they cannot avoid contact they will fight as a defence mechanism.
- Husbandry procedures – Rabbits will often regard their living area as their territory and may show aggressive behaviours towards owners when they are doing normal routine husbandry tasks, that is filling food bowls or changing bedding, thus seeing the owners hand as a threat.
- Un-neutered females – During the spring, which is the rabbit's natural breeding season, females that are not neutered may display aggressive behaviour towards their owner or companions. This behaviour is 'normal' and linked to normal changes in reproductive hormones and should disappear by the end of the summer.
- Pain – Can be a result of a number of diseases (i.e. dental disease) or as a result of incorrect housing leading to spinal deformities and, thus, pain. It is, however, also important to remember that as a prey species rabbits will not show any overt signs of pain and, therefore, aggression towards the owner or other companions could be the only notable sign

5.3.3 Preventing and Minimizing Aggressive Behaviour

There are a number of things that the owner can do with regards to this, including (RWAF, ND):

- Ensuring that rabbits have enough space and environmental enrichment to exercise regularly and also provide stimulation.
- Handling of rabbits from a young age is important in order to ensure that the rabbit is accustomed to people and being handled.
- Rabbits need to like being with people and, as such, some training may be necessary, for example clicker training. However, owners must ensure that they seek advice from someone with a good knowledge of rabbit behaviour and training.
- Never scruff a rabbit and always ensure that good handling techniques are used when picking up and restraining rabbits.
- Neutering of rabbits can help prevent aggressive behaviours associated with reproduction.

Key Points

- The domestic breeds of rabbit demonstrate extensive variation in appearance.
- In more recent years, they have become a very popular children's pet and in the United Kingdom they are the third most popular pet.
- They are one of the most poorly understood species with regards to husbandry and handling.
- It is important that rabbits are socialized from an early age, so that they are able to cope with human interaction and also to different stimuli.
- It is important when handling rabbits that you remain calm at all times, as a prey species rabbits can be startled easily.
- Talking to and stroking the rabbit can help to reduce anxiety and, therefore, ensure that the rabbit is relaxed prior to handling.
- The rabbit's spine must always be supported in a normal position to maintain the normal curvature of the spine at all times to prevent vertebral fractures.
- The hind limbs must always be supported and controlled, as rabbits can cause serious injury and deep wounds to the handler if they kick.
- Do not scruff a rabbit or lift it by its ears.

Self-assessment Questions

1 Which of these methods of restraint is most appropriate for general examination of a rabbit?
   a Towel wrap.
   b Tonic immobilization.
   c Scruffing.
   d Restraint bag.

2 Name two behaviours often shown by aggressive or stressed rabbits.

3 What anatomical considerations should be taken into account when handling rabbits?

4 'Trancing' is a method that has been described for the restraint of rabbits. Under what circumstance might you consider this restraint method and why should it not be used as a general method for restraining rabbits?

References

Bayne, K. (2003) Environmental enrichment of non-human primates, dogs and rabbits used in toxicologic studies. *Toxicology Pathology*, **31** (Suppl), 132–137.

Carneiro, M., Afonso, S., Geraldes, A. *et al.* (2011) The genetic structure of domestic rabbits. *Molecular Biology and Evolution*, **28** (6), 1801–1815.

Dallas, S. (2006) *Animal Biology and Care*, 2nd edn, Blackwell Publishing, Oxford.

Home Office (2015) Annual statistics of scientific procedures on living animals. UK Stationery Office.

Jilge, B. and Hudson, R. (2001) Diversity and development of circadian rhythms in the European rabbit. *Chronobiology International*, **18** (1), 1–26.

McBride, E.A., Day, S., McAdie, T. *et al.* (2006) Trancing rabbits: Relaxed hypnosis or a state of fear? In: Proceedings of the VDWE International Congress on Companion Animal Behaviour and Welfare, Vlaamse Dierenartsenvereniging v.z.w., Sint-Niklaas, Belgium, pp. 135–137 (http://eprints.soton.ac.uk/54860/; last accessed 24 May 2017).

Oxley, J.A, Ellis, C.F, McBride, A. and McCormick, W.D. (2016) A review of handling methods of rabbits within pet, laboratory and veterinary contexts www.ufaw.org.uk/downloads/york-2016—list-of-poster-presentations-23-june.pdf; last accessed 24 May 2017.

PFMA (2015) Pet Population Statistics 2014–2015. Pet Food Manufacturers Association, London (http://www.pfma.org.uk/pet-population-2015; last accessed 24 May 2017).

RSPCA (ND) Rabbit behaviour. http://www.rspca.org.uk/adviceandwelfare/pets/rabbits/behaviour; last accessed 24 May 2017.

RWAF (ND) Hop to it: The RWAF guide to rabbit care. Rabbit Welfare Association and Fund, Tanton, UK. (www.rabbitwelfare.co.uk; last accessed 24 May 2017.)

Schepers, F., Koene, P. and Beerde, B. (2009) Welfare assessment in pet rabbits. *Animal Welfare*, **18**, 477–485.

Wolfensohn, S. and Lloyd, M. (2013) *Handbook of Laboratory Animal Management and Welfare*, 4th edn, John Wiley & Sons Ltd, Chichester.

Further Reading

Ballard, B. and Cheek, R. (2010) *Exotic Animal Medicine for the Veterinary Technician*, 2nd edn, John Wiley & Sons, Inc, Hoboken, NJ.

Girling, S.J. (2013) *Veterinary Nursing of Exotic Pets*, 2nd edn, John Wiley & Sons Ltd, Chichester.

6

Handling and Restraint of Rodents

Bridget Roberts[1] and Stella J. Chapman[2]

[1]*University of Surrey, Guildford, UK*
[2]*University Centre Hartpury, Gloucestershire, UK*

Rodents belong to the order Rodentia and approximately 40% of all mammal species are rodents. There are currently 2277 different species (Wilson and Reeder, 2005). Being one of the most diverse groups of mammals, they are found worldwide on all continents, except Antarctica, and can be found in a variety of habitats.

The term 'companion animal' is used to refer to any pet animal that is kept by humans for companionship and enjoyment. Whilst dogs and cats are regarded as the most popular pets kept in households' worldwide, small mammals, for example rats, hamsters, mice, guinea pigs and so on, are also a popular pet, especially for small children. According to a European survey in 2012, there were approximately 21 250 000 (European Union excluding the Baltic States) and 28 582 000 (Europe) small mammals kept as pets (IFAH, 2012). Rodents are also popular for research; according to UK Home Office statistics, mice accounted for approximately 76% of the total species used for medical research (Home Office, 2014).

6.1 General Species Information

6.1.1 Guinea Pigs

Guinea pigs (*Cavia aperea porcellus*) are also known as 'cavies' and belong to the suborder Hystricomorphs. They were domesticated from the wild cavy approximately 3000–6000 years ago in South America (Stahl, 2003), where they were bred initially for food and were offered as sacrifices by the Incas to their gods. Guinea pigs are now no longer found in the wild and selective breeding has resulted in the many coat colours, patterns and types found today in guinea pigs that are kept as pets. There are three main coat types of guinea pig (Dallas, 2006):

1) smooth or short hair, e.g. Dutch;
2) containing whirls, ridges and rosettes, e.g. Abyssinian;
3) long coated, e.g. Peruvian.

Guinea pigs are also used for research purposes. However, more recently they have been largely replaced by rats and mice in the United Kingdom (Wolfensohn and Lloyd, 2013).

As they are very sociable animals, they should not be kept on their own. Another misconception is that they can be housed with rabbits and this is not the case, as they require a different diet and also are often bullied by rabbits.

6.1.2 Rats

The most common rats, *Rattus norvegicus* (brown rat) and *Rattus* (black rat), are thought to have originated from wetland habitats in Asia. They are found all over the world and are able to adapt to a variety of climates and habitats. They travelled in merchant ships across the world. Rats are used today to clear landmines and for Tuberculosis detection from sputum samples in Africa. White laboratory rats are still used extensively for research, particularly in developing drugs in the medical field.

Around 65 varieties of rat are recognized in the United Kingdom by the National Fancy Rat Society (www.nfrs.org). These are classified into eight sections: self, marked, Russian, shaded, any other varieties (AOV), guide standard varieties, new varieties and Rex and Dumbo (1 group). The most common colours are black, mink, champagne and albino. Hooded rats have a white body with a coloured head. Rats have three coat types (smooth, rex and hairless), which can be combined with any pattern or colour. The Dumbo variety of fancy rat is so called as they have large prominent ears.

6.1.3 Mice

Mice are very adaptable and can be found in a variety of habitats all over the world. Fancy mice and laboratory mice are descended from the *Mus musculus* (house mouse), which is found widely in the wild. Other common species, such as *Apodemus flavicollis* (yellow necked field mouse), *Apodemus sylvaticus* (wood mouse), *Peromyscus municulatus* (deer mouse), *Micromys minutus* (Eurasian harvest mouse) and *Muscardinus avellanarius* (hazel dormouse), can also be found around the world. There are a total of four subgenera and 36 species found around the world and they are one of the most successful mammals due to their ability to adapt and multiply. They are widely kept as pets and used for research due to their small size and ease of breeding.

The National Mouse Club (NMC) (http://www.thenationalmouseclub.co.uk) in the United Kingdom classifies mice into five types: selfs (one solid colour on top, belly and sides), tans (colour on top with rich tan belly), marked (patched with standard colour in combination with white in various patterns), satins (high metallic sheen on coat) and any other variety (AOV), which includes all other mice. Within these groups, over 40 standard varieties are recognized with up to 200 possible colour and coat variations. The most common types are the 'self' variety with a white or black colour.

6.1.4 Hamsters

The Syrian hamster (*Mesocricetus auratus*) is most commonly kept as a domesticated pet and is native to Syria. The first Syrian hamsters were bred in America in 1931 and used in research. They are now endangered in the wild. The name 'hamster' means to hoard in German (hamstern) and the Latin name means 'golden hair'. They are widely available and are very popular as children's pets.

There are four main types of hamster bred in the United Kingdom and recognized by the National Hamster Council (https://hamsters-uk.org). The most common is the

Syrian hamster, which it has many colour varieties and coat types, including long-haired, satin, Rex and short-haired satin. Coat patterns include banded and dominant spot. Dwarf varieties include Russian Campbell and Winter Russian Dwarf hamster (or Siberian, which are not yet found in the UK), Chinese hamster and Robororvski hamster. The largest is the Syrian at 5–6 inches long and the smallest is the Robororvski hamster at 5 cm in length.

6.1.5 Gerbils

Gerbils originated from Mongolia, hence the name Mongolian Gerbil (*Meriones unguiculatus*). They are desert animals found in Africa, India and Asia. Gerbils have only been domesticated in the last 30 years and The National Gerbil Society (NGS) (www.gerbils.co.uk) was founded in 1970 to promote the keeping and showing of gerbils as pets. They were bred in Japan in the 1930s and imported to the USA in 1954, with breeding in the United Kingdom starting in 1964. The *Gerbillinae* group contains more than 100 species of gerbils and Jirds of varying sizes, the largest, the great gerbil (*Rhombomys opimus*), is 15–20 cm long.

The National Gerbil Society classifies gerbils into four categories: selfs, white bellied, any other variety (AOV) and provisional, with over 25 varieties, including albino, black, cinnamon, white spot, dark tailed white, dove and Argente. The most common is the Golden Agouti (sandy colour with dark stripe down the spine and tail).

6.2 Behaviour of Rodents

When animals are domesticated, they will often undergo changes to their bio-behavioural profile, such as reduced aggression and flight behaviours (Price, 1999). For example, the behaviour of the guinea pig has been altered considerably, with domesticated guinea pigs showing less aggression, exploration and orientation behaviour (Künzl and Sachser, 1999). Rodents can be crepuscular (active at dawn and dusk), for example hamsters, diurnal (active both day and night), for example gerbils, or nocturnal (active at night), for example rats and mice.

6.2.1 Anatomical Considerations

- Nocturnal species, for example mice, have enlarged eyes, with some being sensitive to ultraviolet light.
- Many species, for example rats, have long, sensitive whiskers, or vibrissae, for touch.
- Some species, for example hamsters, have cheek pouches, which may be lined with fur.

6.2.2 Social Behaviour

Rodents exhibit a wide range of social behaviours depending on the species, including living in family groups to independent and solitary living. For example:

- Guinea pigs naturally live in breeding groups consisting of one adult male and several females with their offspring. They should always be housed with other guinea pigs, as they form very strong social bonds.

- Rats live in groups of two or more of the same sex. They can be kept as single pets but they tend to do better if housed with one other cage mate. Rats will bond with their human owner.
- Hamsters (of either sex) are better housed singly rather than in groups, as they tend to fight with one another, unless raised since birth.

6.2.3 Communication

In general
- Smell – Rodents use scent marking in many social contexts including inter- and intraspecies communication, in order to mark trails and establish territories. The odour of a predator will depress this behaviour. They are able to recognize close relatives and this allows them to show preferential behaviour (nepotism) toward their kin and also to avoid in-breeding. Hamsters, in particular, become very accustomed to the scent of the group and if one hamster is extensively handled, the group may attack it (Dallas, 2006).
- Vocalization – Many species, particularly those that are diurnal and social, have a wide range of alarm calls. Social species will also have a wider range of vocalizations than solitary species. Many of these vocalizations are at a frequency that humans are unable to hear.

Specific to each species
- *Mice* use pheromones to communicate and it is important to note this when handling mice. Some of the effects of pheromones include (Wolfensohn and Lloyd, 2013):
  - stress in one mouse causes dispersal of other mice;
  - foreign females stimulate aggression by other females;
  - group housed females become anoestrus and resume normal oestrus behaviour if a male is introduced;
  - coexisting males emit pheromones to reduce aggression within the group, but which cause foreign males to avoid the territory.
- *Gerbils* communicate through thumping their hind legs in order to indicate dominance or to warn of danger.
- *Guinea pigs* are neophobic and mistrust new food or changes to normal routine. Therefore, it is very important to handle young guinea pigs on a regular basis and expose them to a variety of foods. Guinea pigs use a repertoire of up to eleven vocalisations to communicate (Table 6.1).

6.3 Handling and Restraint of Small Rodents

6.3.1 General Guidelines

The following points are provided as general guidance for handling of all the smaller rodents, that is mice, hamsters and gerbils.

- Ensure that the area is safe and secure.
- Prepare baskets with substrate, open lid for transport next to cage or prepare a non-slip surface for examination with a small towel for restraint.

Table 6.1 Guinea pig vocalizations.

Vocalization	Meaning
Chut	Exploring
Chutter/Rumble	Dominance/Mating
Whine	Unhappy/Uncomfortable
Whistle	Calling/Excitement
Drrr	Fear
Tweet/Chirp	Startled
Scream	Pain/Fear/Distress
Squeal/Wheeking	Excitement
Purr	Content

- Remain calm and quiet.
- Observe the animal's behaviour in the enclosure and observe for aggressive behaviour.
- Talk to the animal quietly upon approach to the cage to alert to your presence.
- Rub some substrate between your hands to aid handling (Figure 6.1).
- Ensure the animal is awake prior to approach or you may be bitten.
- Once the animal is awake, offer a closed fist and allow sniffing to take place whilst talking. Be aware that most rodents have poor eyesight in daylight and may bite if startled.
- Approach from the side as they are prey animals and grasping from above will mimic being captured, unless handled regularly.

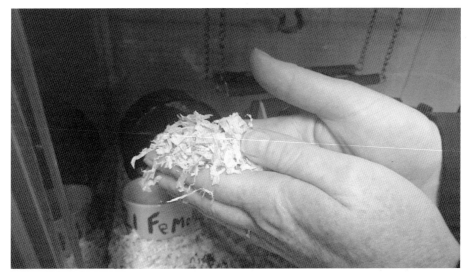

Figure 6.1 Rubbing substrate on hands prior to handling.

6.3.2 Points to Consider

The following points regarding rodents in general should be noted:

- It is important to note that they are obligate nasal breathers and care must be taken to avoid blocking the nostrils during restraint.
- Care should be taken not to grasp tightly around the chest to allow for normal respiration.
- Rodents have protruding eye globes and poor handling or covering with a towel may cause injury.
- Tail base grasping may result in tail sloughing and should be avoided. The tail may be grasped very gently to aid restraint; however, tail restraint has been shown to cause anxiety and discomfort.
- Rodents will jump and should always be restrained on a table.
- Scruffing is rarely necessary except in aggressive animals or for medical procedures.

6.3.3 Mice

Figures 6.2 and 6.3 demonstrate how to use tube capture with a mouse to aid capture and restraint. This method can greatly reduce the stress associated with handling mice and is highly recommended.

6.3.4 Hamsters and Gerbils

Handling of hamsters and gerbils follow the same general principles. Figure 6.4 demonstrates restraint of a gerbil.

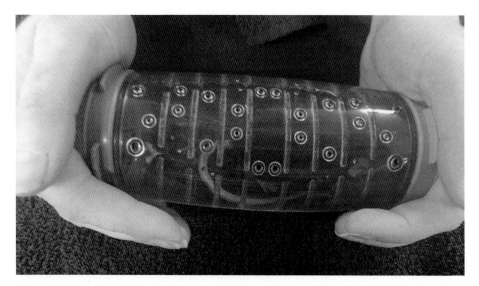

Figure 6.2 Tube capture (Source: Courtesy of Brinsbury Campus, Chichester College).

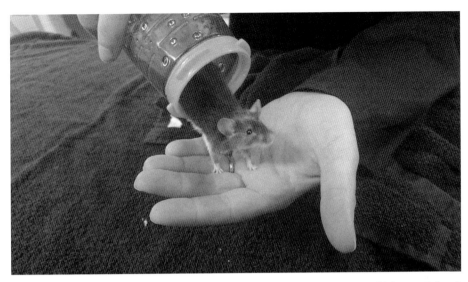

Figure 6.3 Release from tube capture (Source: Courtesy of Brinsbury Campus, Chichester College).

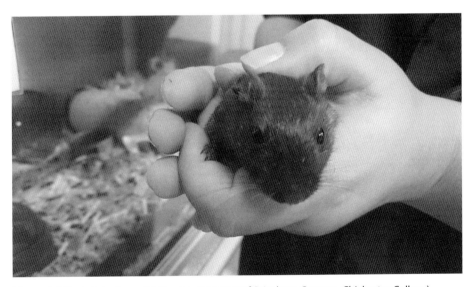

Figure 6.4 Restraint of a gerbil (Source: Courtesy of Brinsbury Campus, Chichester College).

Approach
Step 1 – Approach calmly with two hands (Figure 6.5).
Step 2 – Scoop with both hands from underneath and cup in the hands (Figure 6.6).
Step 3 – Alternatively, use cup/tube or house to lift (Figure 6.7).

General table restraint
Place the hamster on the table with the handler's index and middle fingers placed over the shoulders, and the remaining fingers restraining the body (Figure 6.8).

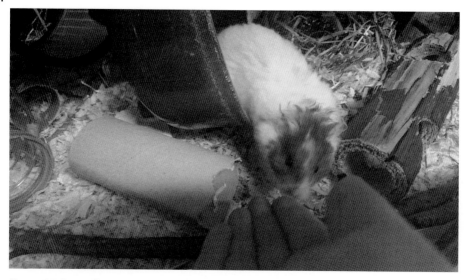

Figure 6.5 Step 1 for capturing hamsters and gerbils (Source: Courtesy of Brinsbury Campus, Chichester College).

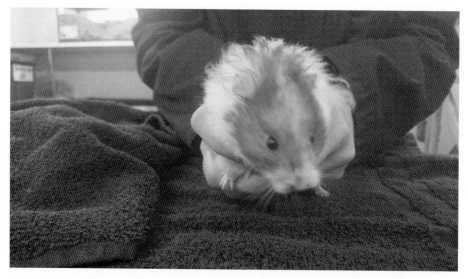

Figure 6.6 Step 2 for capturing hamsters and gerbils (Source: Courtesy of Brinsbury Campus, Chichester College).

Restraint for sexing or examination of the abdomen

Grasp the hamster over the shoulders with the handler's thumb and little finger behind the forelegs. Lift and support the hindquarters with the other hand. Turn over gently, supporting the hindquarters (Figure 6.9).

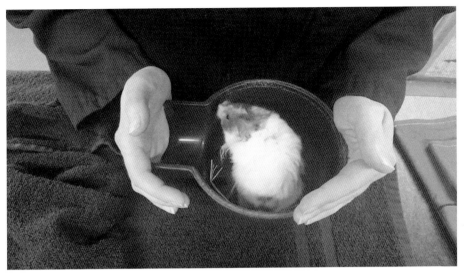

Figure 6.7 Step 3 for capturing hamsters and gerbils (Source: Courtesy of Brinsbury Campus, Chichester College).

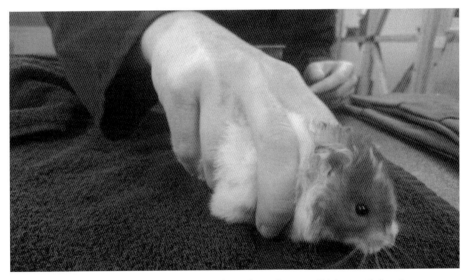

Figure 6.8 Table restraint (Source: Courtesy of Brinsbury Campus, Chichester College).

Restraint for aggressive hamsters

Scruffing may be necessary for aggressive hamsters. The handler's thumb and forefingers grasp the loose skin over the shoulders, whilst the remaining fingers support the hamsters' bodyweight and the other hand supports the hindquarters (Figure 6.10).

Scruffing may cause the eyes to prolapse. It is, therefore, important not to scruff directly at the back of the neck in order to avoid this.

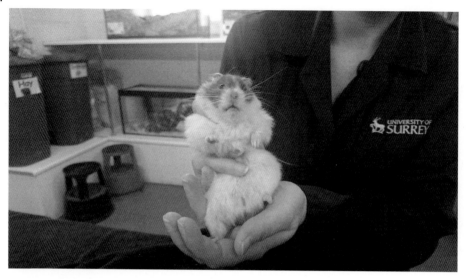

Figure 6.9 Restraint for examination of the abdomen (Source: Courtesy of Brinsbury Campus, Chichester College).

It is important to note that aggression is more common in the smaller breeds, for example Roborovrski and Chinese. The larger Syrian hamster is generally more friendly and easier to handle due to its larger size.

6.4   Handling and Restraint of Rats

6.4.1   Approach (Figure 6.11)

Prepare the basket with a lid for transport or a non-slip surface for examination.

- Remain calm and quiet.
- Observe animal behaviour in enclosure, observe for aggressive behaviour.
- Talk to animal quietly upon approach to cage to alert to your presence.
- Rub some substrate between hands to aid handling.
- Ensure animal is awake prior to approach or you may be bitten.
- Once awake, offer closed fist and allow sniffing whilst talking.

6.4.2   Capture

Open your hand and the rat may walk into cupped hands. If not, cup and scoop up the rat with both hands from underneath. Hands must close as rodents will jump. Alternatively, allow the rat to climb into a tunnel or cup and occlude both ends with your hands.

6.4.3   General Table Restraint

Grasp the rat over the shoulders, with thumb and little finger behind the forelegs. Lift and support the hindquarters with the other hand. Place the rat on the table with the

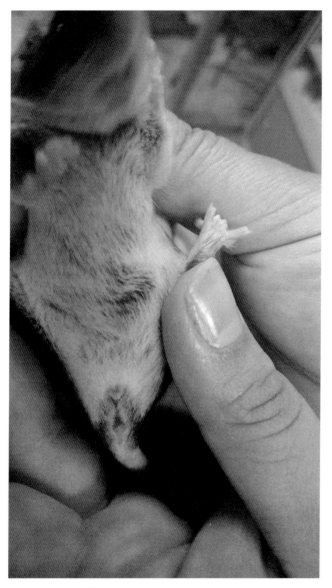

Figure 6.10 Scruffing of an aggressive hamster (Source: Courtesy of Brinsbury Campus, Chichester College).

index and middle fingers over the shoulders and remaining fingers restraining the body (Figure 6.12).

6.4.4 Restraint for Sexing or Examination of the Abdomen

Follow the same initial procedure as for general table restraint. Then gently turn the rat over, supporting the hindquarters (Figure 6.13).

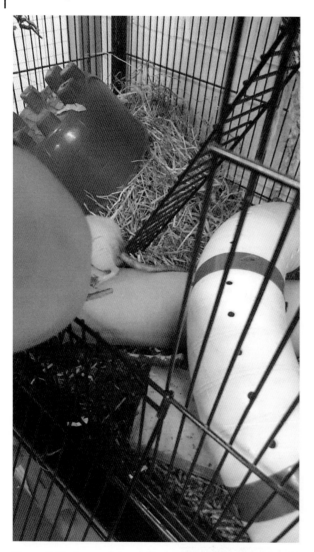

Figure 6.11 Approach to rat (Source: Courtesy of Brinsbury Campus, Chichester College).

6.4.5 Additional Methods of Restraint

Additional restraint can be applied by using the thumb under the mandible to prevent biting. Scruffing is rarely necessary and causes stress. Other methods such as a towel wrap or examination in a tube are simple and less stressful for the rat

It is important to note that rats are obligate nasal breathers and care must be taken to avoid blocking the nostrils during restraint. Care should also be taken not to grasp tightly around the chest to allow for normal respiration.

Tail base grasping may result in the tail sloughing and should be avoided. The tail may be grasped very gently to aid restraint. However, tail restraint has been shown to cause anxiety and discomfort.

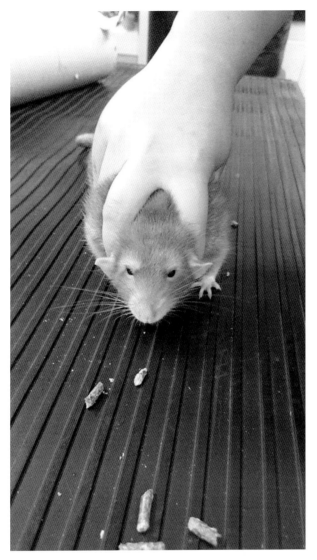

Figure 6.12 Table restraint (Source: Courtesy of Brinsbury Campus, Chichester College).

6.4.6 Aggression

Rats are usually very friendly and rarely bite, but may bite if scared or woken suddenly. Signs of aggression include:

- stiffening of the body;
- arching the back;
- hairs may stand on end;
- tail wagging;
- body shaking;
- they may stand on hind limbs and box;
- may vocalize by long squeak, or squeal or hiss in protest;

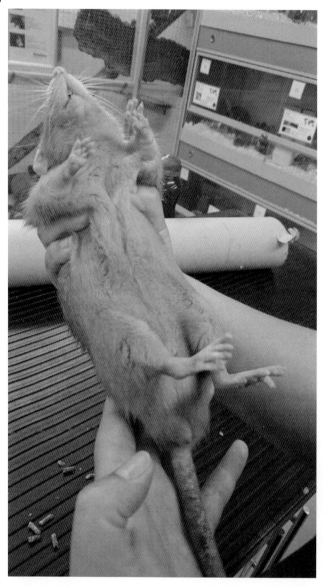

Figure 6.13 Restraint for examination of the abdomen (Source: Courtesy of Brinsbury Campus, Chichester College).

6.5 Handling and Restraint of Guinea Pigs

6.5.1 Approach

Approach in a confident manner, from the front and bend down to the guinea pigs level. Spend a moment talking and stroking to the guinea until they are relaxed (Figure 6.14).

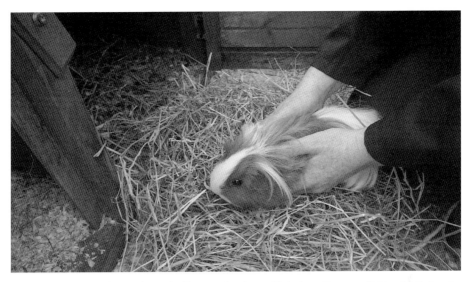

Figure 6.14 Approach to guinea pig (Source: Courtesy of Brinsbury Campus, Chichester College).

6.5.2 Capture

Allow the guinea pig to climb into a tunnel or house and occlude both ends with your hands.

Step 1 – Place one hand over the shoulders and cover the eyes to calm the guinea pig (Figure 6.15). Then move one hand under the chest behind the forelegs. Spend time gently stroking and covering the eyes to minimize stress.

Step 2 – Once calm, lift the guinea pig by supporting the hindquarters (Figure 6.16).

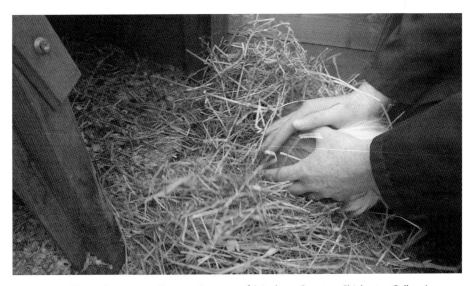

Figure 6.15 Step 1 for capture (Source: Courtesy of Brinsbury Campus, Chichester College).

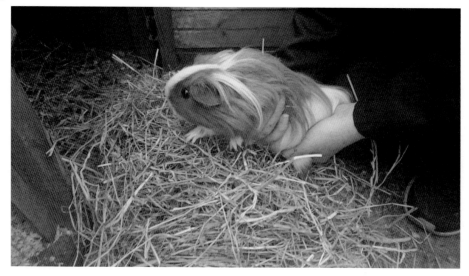

Figure 6.16 Step 2 for capture (Source: Courtesy of Brinsbury Campus, Chichester College).

6.5.3 General Table Restraint

Step 1 – Place the guinea pig on a table with the head tucked into the elbow and the hands and arms wrapped around the guinea pigs body (Figure 6.17).

Step 2 – Place one hand over the back and the other hand over the eyes, this will prevent the guinea pig from moving forward (Figure 6.18).

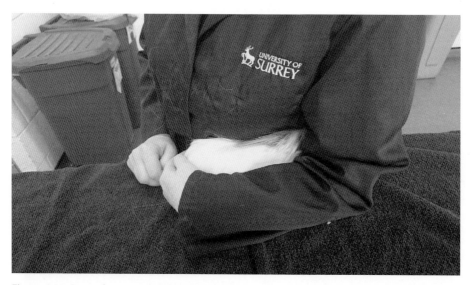

Figure 6.17 Step 1 for general table restraint (Source: Courtesy of Brinsbury Campus, Chichester College).

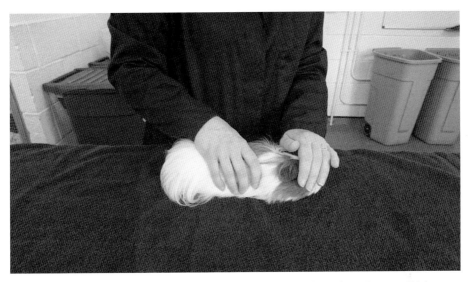

Figure 6.18 Step 2 for general table restraint (Source: Courtesy of Brinsbury Campus, Chichester College).

Step 3 – Place the guinea pig on the table with the head facing away from the handler with the handlers thumbs placed over the shoulders, with the index fingers in front of the forelegs and the fingers wrapped around the chest (Figure 6.19).

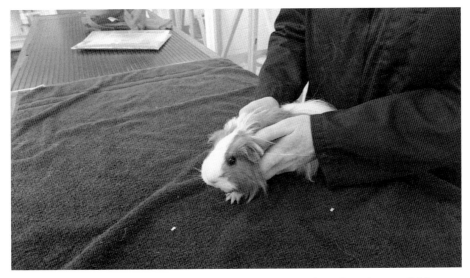

Figure 6.19 Step 3 for general table restraint (Source: Courtesy of Brinsbury Campus, Chichester College).

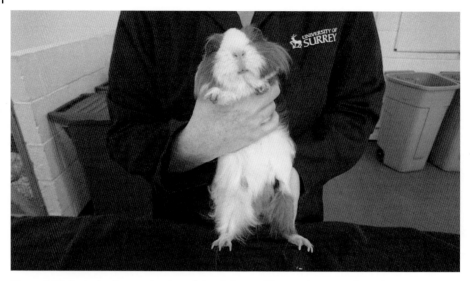

Figure 6.20 Restraint for examination of the abdomen (Source: Courtesy of Brinsbury Campus, Chichester College).

6.5.4   Restraint for Sexing or Examination of the Abdomen

Place one hand under the chest and grasp the forelimbs between the handlers thumb and fingers with one hand. Place the other hand around the hindquarters. Then gently lift and place the guinea pig against the handler's chest (Figure 6.20).

6.5.5   Carrying a Guinea Pig

Step 1 – Hold the guinea pig under the chest, behind the forelimbs with one hand and hold around the hindquarters with the other hand (Figure 6.21).
Step 2 – Gently turn the guinea pig to rest in the handler's forearm and tuck the head under the elbow. Place the other hand on top of the guinea pig for extra security (Figure 6.22).

6.5.6   Aggression in Guinea Pigs

Aggressive behaviour is fairly rare, as guinea pigs are normally very docile. However, they can become aggressive during the breeding season, or due to a lack of handling, or poor handling. Signs of aggression include:

- lunging;
- baring teeth;
- biting;
- head tossing;
- strutting;
- scratching;
- vocalization, including 'rumble', 'drr', or 'scream';

Guinea pigs can inflict very serious injuries, particularly deep scratches or bites. These guinea pigs are best handled in a large towel.

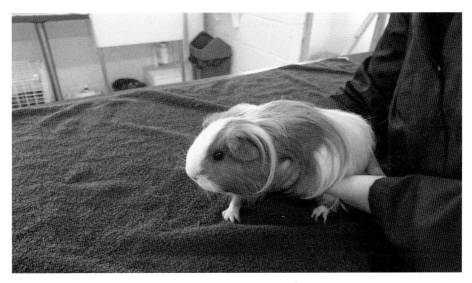

Figure 6.21 Step 1 for carrying a guinea pig (Source: Courtesy of Brinsbury Campus, Chichester College).

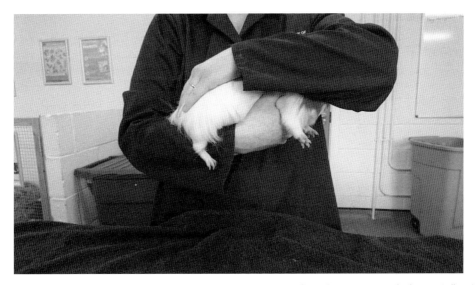

Figure 6.22 Step 2 for carrying a guinea pig (Source: Courtesy of Brinsbury Campus, Chichester College).

Key Points

- Rodents belong to the order Rodentia; approximately 40% of all mammal species are rodents.
- Guinea pigs are very sociable animals and should not be kept on their own.
- Around 65 varieties of rat are recognized in the United Kingdom by the National Fancy Rat Society.

- Fancy mice and laboratory mice are descended from the *Mus musculus* (house mouse), which are found widely in the wild.
- Rodents can be crepuscular (active at dawn and dusk), such as hamsters, diurnal (active both day and night), such as gerbils, or nocturnal (active at night), such as rats and mice.
- Hamsters (of either sex) are better housed singly rather than in groups, as they tend to fight with one another, unless raised since birth.
- Many rodent species, particularly those that are diurnal and social, have a wide range of alarm calls.
- Guinea pigs use a repertoire of up to eleven vocalizations to communicate.
- Mice use pheromones to communicate and it is important to note this when handling them.
- Observe the animal's behaviour in the enclosure and observe for aggressive behaviour.
- Ensure the animal is awake prior to approach or you may be bitten.
- Rub some substrate between your hands to aid handling.
- Rodents will jump and should always be restrained on a table.
- Tail base grasping may result in the tail sloughing and should be avoided.

Self-assessment Questions

1 Which of the following is *not* a normal guinea pig behaviour?
   a Popcorning
   b Strutting
   c Head Tossing
   d Thumping

2 Which rodent species is *not* at risk to deglove the tail when handled?
   a Rat
   b Gerbil
   c Hamster
   d Mouse

3 Define the terms (i) crepuscular, (ii) nocturnal and (iii) diurnal and state which rodents belong in which category

4 Discuss how rodents use smell to communicate?

5 For which species of rodent may scruffing be considered necessary and why?

Answers can be found in the back of the book.

References

Dallas, S. (2006) *Animal Biology and Care*, 2nd edn, Blackwell Publishing, Oxford.
IFAH (2012) European Pet Food Industry: Facts and Figures. International Federation for Animal Health, Brussels (http://www.ifaheurope.org/companion-animals/about-pets.html; last accessed 25 May 2017).

Home Office (2014) 2013 Animal Research Statistics from the Home Office. http://www .understandinganimalresearch.org.uk/news/communications-media/2013-animal-research-statistics-from-the-home-office/; last accessed 25 May 2017.

Künzl, C. and Sachser, N. (1999) The behavioral endocrinology of domestication: a comparison between the domestic guinea pig (*Cavia aperea f. porcellus*) and its wild ancestor, the cavy (*Cavia aperea*). *Hormones and Behavior*, **35** (1), 28–37. doi: 10.1006/ hbeh.1998.1493.

Price, E.O. (1999) Behavioural development in animals undergoing domestication. *Applied Animal Behaviour Science*, **65** (3), 245–271. doi: 10.1016/S0168-1591(99)00087-8.

Stahl, P.W. (2003) Pre-Columbian Andean animal domesticates at the edge of empire. *World Archaeology*, **34** (3), 470–483. doi: 10.1080/0043824021000026459.

Wilson, D.E. and Reeder, D.M. (2005) *Mammal Species of the World: A Taxonomic and Geographic Reference*, 3rd edn, Johns Hopkins University Press, Baltimore, MD.

Wolfensohn, S. and Lloyd, M. (2013) *Handbook of Laboratory Animal Management and Welfare*, 4th edn, John Wiley & Sons Ltd, Chichester.

Further Reading

Ballard, B. and Cheek, R. (2010) *Exotic Animal Medicine for the Veterinary Technician*, 2nd edn, John Wiley & Sons, Inc, Hoboken, NJ.

Girling, S.J. (2013) *Veterinary Nursing of Exotic Pets*, 2nd edn, John Wiley & Sons Ltd, Chichester.

7

Handling and Restraint of Ferrets

Bridget Roberts[1] and Stella J. Chapman[2]

[1]University of Surrey, Guildford, UK
[2]University Centre Hartpury, Gloucestershire, UK

Ferrets (*Mustela putorius furo*) belong to the family Mustelidae. It is believed that ferrets were first domesticated some 2000 years ago in countries of Southern Europe, bordering the Mediterranean, where they were bred specifically for hunting rabbits. They are carnivores and their nearest wild relative is thought to be the European polecat. Ferrets still continue to be used for hunting rabbits in the United Kingdom as well as for pest control and are a popular domestic pet, with an estimation of more than 100 000 kept in the United Kingdom alone (Vinke and Schoemaker, 2012).

Commercial breeding of ferrets has resulted in a number of different breeds recognized by differences in coat colour; they include the:

- Albino (English) ferret.
- Sable or fitch ferret (black guard hair).
- Siamese ferret (brown guard hair).
- Silver mitt ferret (sable with white chest and feet).
- Black-footed ferret (endangered species in North America).

A healthy ferret can live up to 10 years of age, with the average lifespan being approximately six years.

7.1 Behaviour of Ferrets

The word ferret is taken from the Latin '*furonem*' and the Italian '*furone*', meaning thief; with the connotations of the verb describing the ferret's behaviour and traits as: 'to remove from a hiding place, search out with keenness or draw out by shrewd questioning'.

Wild ferrets are largely solitary (Clapperton, 2001); domesticated ferrets, however, are sociable and usually enjoy living in groups. If socialized and well-handled from an early age, ferrets can form strong bonds with their owners. Frequent handling of ferrets as well as neutering prior to puberty (approximately six months) helps to minimize aggressive behaviour.

In the wild ferrets spend a large proportion of their time foraging and have wide home ranges, thus ferrets are naturally very active. They are intelligent and thus need mental as

Safe Handling and Restraint of Animals: A Comprehensive Guide, First Edition. Stella J. Chapman.
© 2018 John Wiley & Sons Ltd. Published 2018 by John Wiley & Sons Ltd.

well as physical stimulation; this is very important in young ferrets, as play is required for them to develop motor and social skills, in addition to learning and predatory behaviours (Spinka *et al.*, 2001). Good socialization is very important for ferrets in order to prepare them to live in a human environment. Handlers need to understand that ferrets are (Vinke and Schoemaker, 2012):

- highly motivated and need to explore and forage;
- they require adequate resting opportunities and play opportunities;
- social organization of groups is important in order to decrease interspecies and territorial aggression.

7.1.1   Communication

As with other species, ferrets use a number of different methods to communicate with each other and also to communicate a range of emotions (Lloyd, 2013).

- Vocalization – Ferrets produce a variety of different noises, such as hiss and chuckle (playing), scream (fighting, frightened or threatened) and grumble (foraging).
- Vision – Ferrets have relatively poor vision and, as a consequence of this, their natural instinct is to nip at objects that move in their field of vision. This is important for handlers to be aware of as they may bite if they do not see what is in front of them.
- Scent – Ferrets are carnivores and use smell to hunt. They also use scent to communicate with each other.

7.2   Handling and Restraint of Ferrets

7.2.1   General points

- Ensure that personal protective clothing (PPE) is worn by the handler in order to reduce the incidence of allergens and zoonotic disease.
- Prepare either a basket (with a lid) for transport, or a non-slip surface for examination.
- Remain calm and quiet.
- Observe ferret behaviour whilst they are in the enclosure and, in particular, note any aggressive behaviour.
- Talk to the animal quietly upon approach to the cage in order to alert the ferret to your presence.
- Rub some substrate between your hands as this will aid handling.
- Ensure that the animal is awake prior to approach, or you may be bitten.
- If the animal is awake, offer a closed fist and allow the ferret to sniff your hand whilst you are talking.

7.2.2   Approach (Figure 7.1)

A calm and quiet approach is essential. As previously mentioned, ensure that the ferret is awake and attempt to gently stroke the ferret. Due to the fact that ferrets have poor vision, be careful when offering a hand for a ferret to sniff. Also, as they are carnivores, ensure that the handlers PPE has not previously been worn to handle other species such

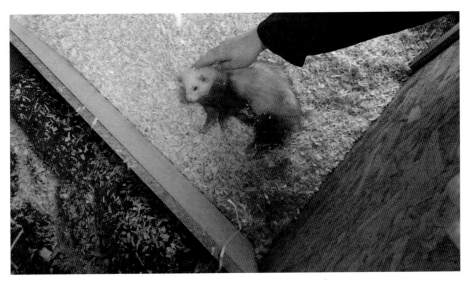

Figure 7.1 Approach to a ferret (Source: Courtesy of Brinsbury Campus, Chichester College).

as rabbits. Ferrets would naturally prey upon rabbits and may nip at the smell of them on hands or clothing.

7.2.3 Capture

There are two options for capture.

Option 1 – Allow the ferret to climb into a tunnel and occlude both ends with your hands.

Option 2 – Grasp over the shoulders and gently lift whilst supporting the hind limbs (Figure 7.2).

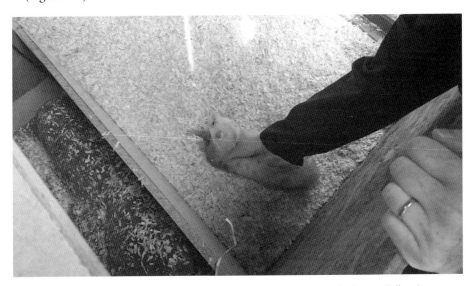

Figure 7.2 Capture Option 2 (Source: Courtesy of Brinsbury Campus, Chichester College).

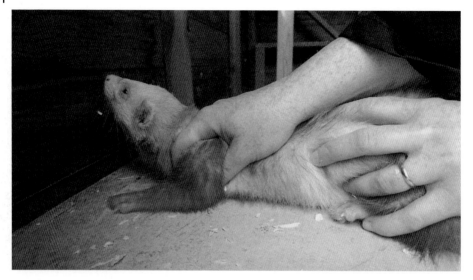

Figure 7.3 Table restraint (Source: Courtesy of Brinsbury Campus, Chichester College).

7.2.4   General Table Restraint

Put the ferret on a table with the handler's index and middle fingers placed over the ferret's shoulders and the handler's remaining fingers restraining the ferret's body. The handler's thumb should be behind the ferret's elbow to prevent the ferret from moving backwards. The handler's other hand should be placed over the hindquarters to provide extra restraint (Figure 7.3).

7.2.5   Restraint for Sexing and Examination of the Abdomen

The ferret should be grasped as above and then gently lifted using the other hand to support the hindquarters (Figure 7.4). The thumb may be placed under the mandible to prevent biting in more aggressive animals.

7.2.6   Restraint of Aggressive Ferrets

Aggressive ferrets may be handled with gauntlets (Figure 7.5) to prevent injury to the handler. Ferrets may also be scruffed if necessary. Many procedures can be performed by distracting the ferret with high quality cat food, fed on a tongue depressor. This will enable the handler to perform tasks such as nail clips and physical examination.

7.2.7   Use of Harnesses

There are a number of harness available that allow owners/handlers to take their ferret for a walk. Numerous websites are available with advice on how to train a ferret to walk on a harness. At present, however, there is no scientific research available on the safe use of harnesses and whether walking a ferret using this device has any positive or negative effects on the wellbeing of ferrets.

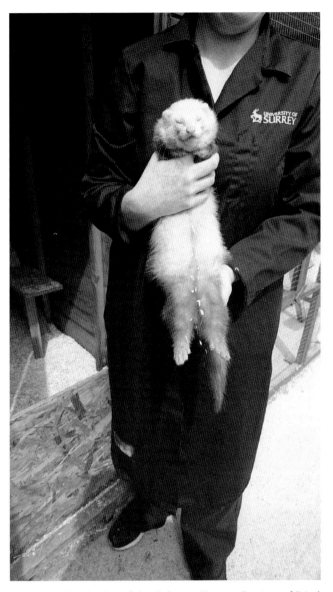

Figure 7.4 Examination of the abdomen (Source: Courtesy of Brinsbury Campus, Chichester College).

Key Points

- Ferrets are carnivores and their nearest wild relative is thought to be the European polecat.
- Commercial breeding of ferrets has resulted in a number of different breeds recognized by differences in coat colour.
- The word ferret is taken from the Latin '*furonem*' and the Italian '*furone*', meaning thief.

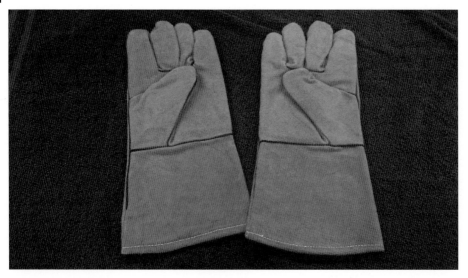

Figure 7.5 Gauntlets.

- Frequent handling of ferrets as well as neutering prior to puberty (approximately 6 months) helps to minimize aggressive behaviour.
- Good socialization is very important for ferrets in order to prepare them to live in a human environment.
- As with other species, ferrets use a number of different methods to communicate with each other and also to communicate a range of emotions.
- Due to the fact that ferrets have poor vision, be careful when offering a hand for a ferret to sniff.

Self-assessment Questions

1   Discuss the ways in which ferrets communicate?

2   Why is it important that ferrets are socialized from an early age?

3   Describe how you would handle a ferret on a table for examination?

4   Describe how you would restrain an aggressive ferret?

Answers can be found in the back of the book.

References

Clapperton, B.K. (2001) Advances in New Zealand mammalogy 1990–2000: feral ferret. *Journal of the Royal Society of New Zealand*, **31**, 185–203.
Lloyd, M. (2013) Housing and husbandry of ferrets, NC3Rs, London (https://www.nc3rs. org.uk/3rs-resources/housing-and-husbandry/ferrets; last accessed 26 May 2017).

Spinka, M., Newberry, R.C. and Bekoff, M. (2001) Mammalian play: Training for the unexpected. *The Quarterly Review of Biology*, **76** (2), 141–168.

Vinke, C.M. and Schoemaker, N.J. (2012) The welfare of ferrets (*Mustela putorius furo*): A review of housing and management of pet ferrets. *Applied Animal Behaviour*, **139**, 155–168.

Further Reading

Fisher, P.G. (2006) Ferret behaviour. In: *Exotics Pet Behaviour. Birds, Reptiles, and Small Mammals* (eds T.B. Bays, T. Lightfoot, J. Mayer), Saunders, MO.

Fox, J.G and Marini, R.P. (2014) *Biology and Diseases of the Ferret*, 3rd edn, John Wiley & Sons Ltd, Chichester.

Hubrecht, R. and Kirkwood, J. (eds) (2010) *The UFAW Handbook on the Care and Management of Laboratory and Other Research Animals*, 8th edn, John Wiley & Sons Ltd, Chichester.

8

Handling and Restraint of Horses and Donkeys

Stella J. Chapman[1] and Krista M. McLennan[2]

[1]University Centre Hartpury, Gloucestershire, UK
[2]Chester University, Chester, UK

The evolutionary ancestor of the modern horse is known as *Hyracotherium*, or the more commonly used term of *Eohippus* (the dawn horse), and fossils found in both North America and Europe depict an animal that stood 4.2–5 hands, with padded feet and teeth that indicated a diet mainly adapted to that of a browser. The subsequent evolution of the horse took place mainly in North America and much of the evolutionary history is based on changes to the physical appearance of the horse, until the end of the Pliocene period when *Equus* (the genus to which all horses, donkeys and zebras belong) evolved. The wild horse (*Equus ferus*) was first tamed by inhabitants of the Eurasian Steppes between 4000 and 6000 years ago (Cohen, 2012) and with the advent of domestication the term *Equus caballus* was used, with the modern horse being found widespread across central Asia and most of Europe. Again, as with many of the species mentioned in this book, the question of whether domestication took place in a single location or in multiple areas remains controversial.

With regards to the horse, there are many ways in which it is possible to trace a timeline of domestication events. The earliest archaeological evidence of human–horse interaction can be found in cave paintings in France and Spain, painted around 15 000 years ago when horses were hunted for their meat and hides (Goodwin, 1999). From that time the manner in which horses were used by humans' moves from being a food source, to draught animal, war horse and then to the advent of the modern horse, which has many roles in society, including that of a companion. With domestication, natural selection has, on the whole, been replaced by artificial selection, whereby humans control access to food, shelter and potential mates and, thus, have a direct impact on the breeds.

According to a report published by the Food and Agriculture Organization of the United Nations in 2006, the total global equine population was estimated to be 58 million, with the USA having the highest number of horses (Horsetalk, 2007). Horse population statistics are not easy to find; however, the horse is one of the most popular domesticated species that humans like to own. There are very few statistics available on the number of injuries associated with handling horses. Whilst the majority of injuries to humans in their association with horses is caused due to riding accidents, one study that looked at equestrian injuries over a five year period in Canada reported that 30–40% of injuries

Safe Handling and Restraint of Animals: A Comprehensive Guide, First Edition. Stella J. Chapman.
© 2018 John Wiley & Sons Ltd. Published 2018 by John Wiley & Sons Ltd.

occurred to people on the ground, near the horse (Sorli, 2000). A more recent study in Australia that looked at the incidence of injuries caused by horses to veterinary and animal science students concluded that injury on the ground is common and a proactive approach to injury prevention is recommended for people who handle horses (Riley *et al.*, 2015).

The donkey (*Equus asinus*) descended from the wild African ass (*E. africanus*) in north-eastern Africa some 6000 years ago. Two subspecies of ass, namely the Nubian ass and Somali ass are thought to have had a role in the characteristic traits of the modern donkey, although recent mitochondrial DNA suggests that the only the Nubian ass contributed genetically to the domestic donkey (Kimura *et al.*, 2013). Both these subspecies of ass are listed on the IUCN Red List as critically endangered (Moehlman *et al.*, 2015). The earliest archaeological evidence of the domesticated donkey dates back to 4600–4000 BC near Cairo, Egypt (Rossel *et al.*, 2008).

Over 95% of donkeys are kept specifically as 'work animals', with their most common role being as a means of transport or pack animal. It is estimated that there are some 44 million donkeys worldwide, with a further population of some 15 million mules being kept (Starkey and Starkey, 1998). Whilst donkeys are found worldwide, the majority of them are in developing countries.

For the purpose of this chapter, discussion points refer to equids as a group and any key discussion points that distinguish differences between horses and donkeys are highlighted in the relevant section.

8.1 Equine Behaviour

As with many of the other large mammals discussed in this book, equids are social animals that prefer to associate with their own kind but will also accept other species as companions. The idea being that 'safety in numbers' is the best strategy for survival. Flight is the main defence tool that horses use when faced with a threat. However, aggressive behaviour is also a normal behaviour shown by stallions and also by mares with foals at foot in a given situation. What is unique about our relationship with the horse (and donkey), unlike other domesticated species, is that we ride them and this fact lends itself to a special bond between the horse and the rider. It must be stated at this point that the emphasis on handling horses for the purpose of this book is with regards to handling from the ground.

Whilst equine vision is inferior to that of humans with regards to colour recognition and depth perception (due to the lateral position of the eyes) the horse is better equipped with regards to night vision, peripheral vision and in the speed of accommodation, which is accomplished by altering head position (Miller, 2006). Thus, their reaction time is far superior to many other domesticated species and this quick reaction (especially to novel objects) can mean that many horses react by jumping (spooking) away from the 'frightening' object.

8.1.1 Temperament

It is interesting when discussing the behaviour of horses that the word 'temperament' is often used. According to the Oxford English Dictionary, temperament is defined as '*an animal's nature, especially as it permanently affects their behaviour'*. Many owners and trainers of horses will state that assessing a horse's temperament is important for breeding and performance; however, there is currently no recognized standard method available for temperament assessment (McGreevy, 2004).

8.1.2 Communication

In order to understand behaviour it is important that we recognize how equids communicate. As with other species, a number of means of communication are employed and it is important when handling equids that we can at least interpret some of the more obvious communication signals. The main methods that equids use to communicate are summarized in Table 8.1.

Figures 8.1 and 8.2 depict horses that are demonstrating a relaxed posture whilst in the stable environment. Figure 8.1 shows a horse with the hind foot flexed, which is a normal resting position of horses; horses will generally alternate between resting the hind feet. The horse also has the ears to one side and the head in a relaxed position. Figure 8.2

Table 8.1 Methods of equid communication (Source: Houpt, 2011. Reproduced with permission of John Wiley & Sons).

Method	Description
Vocalizations	
Neigh (whinny)	A greeting or separation call used for herd cohesion. Some horses will call to their owners but only when they are in their line of sight.
Nicker	Care-giving or care-soliciting call – most often seen between a mare and her foal.
Snorts, squeals and roars	Roar is a high-amplitude vocalization made by a stallion and is usually directed at a mare; a sharp snort is an alarm call; more prolonged snorting or sneezing snorts are associated with frustration; squeals are a defensive greeting heard frequently when horses are forming a dominance hierarchy; a squeal may also be a response to pain.
Visual signals	
Expression	Ear position is the most common emotional indicator in equids, for example an alert horse will look directly at the object of interest with the ears held forward, whereas ears that are flattened against the head are a sign of aggression. Other facial expressions are more subtle and have been the focus of recent research, especially with regards response to pain.
Posture	A horse that is relaxed will stand quietly; frustration can be shown by pawing the ground; tail lashing and pawing can be signs of discomfort.
Tactile sense	Horses are very sensitive to pressure and touch on the skin; this has been used by humans with regards to the use of the twitch where pressure is placed on the upper lip.
Olfactory signals	
Scent marking	Most important for sexual behaviour, that is flehmen response by stallions

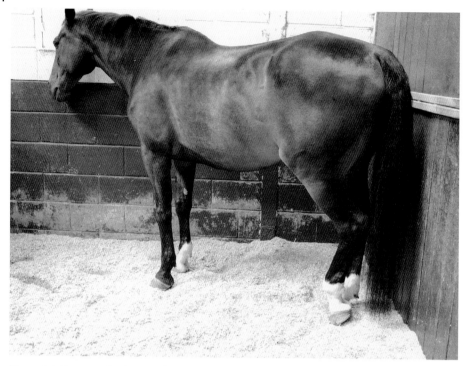

Figure 8.1 Horse resting in a stable (Source: Courtesy of Brinsbury Campus, Chichester College).

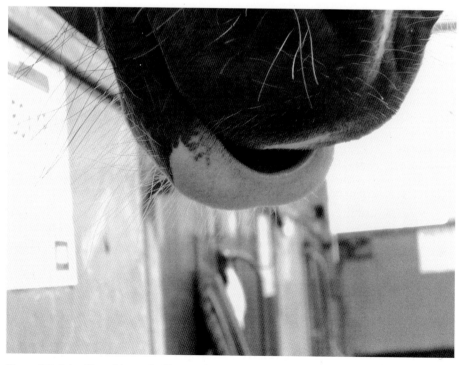

Figure 8.2 Relaxation of lower lip (Source: Courtesy of Brinsbury Campus, Chichester College).

shows a horse with the bottom lip drooping, which is another behaviour sign commonly associated with a relaxed horse.

8.1.3 Key Differences Between Horses and Donkeys

Many books that have been written about the behaviour of equids focus on the behaviour of horses. Therefore, whilst the section above has discussed equine behaviour in general, in this section focus will be given to the key differences with regards to donkey behaviour.

8.1.3.1 In General

Wild (feral) donkeys come from very arid regions where they are less likely to find food and water. This means they tend to live in much smaller groups than wild (feral) horses and many lead solitary lives. Donkeys living in these areas are known to be territorial, defending their very limited resources.

Donkeys do not overtly express signs of pain or stress but are more subtle in their signals. This is especially when compared to horses. They **do not** have a different threshold level, however. This is a very important behaviour to be aware of when handling and restraining donkeys. Observe for the subtle signs that something might be wrong and give the donkey time to show you.

Donkeys form very strong bonds with their field companions (Murray *et al.*, 2013) and this relationship is very important to them. Donkeys prefer to be with their own kind (Proops *et al.*, 2012) but will bond with other equids, such as horses, mules and hinnies, if this is all that is available to them. Social bonds between donkeys and their handlers or carers are also important, and donkeys are very friendly towards people they know but very wary of anyone unfamiliar.

Mules and hinnies (crosses between donkeys and horses) take behaviour from both parents. It is important to understand both donkey and horse behaviour.

8.1.3.2 How Donkey Behaviour Can Affect Handling

Living in smaller groups or as an individual, means that as a prey animal fleeing is not the best strategy to escape a predator. This makes donkeys less likely to flee from a situation, but stand still and study it before reacting. Because they are less likely to flee, when restricted they are more likely to try to fight. This behaviour of standing still or being aggressive whilst restrained is often confused with stubbornness.

Donkeys may have been handled much less than most horses, as they are often an unridden companion for another equid, or a guard animal for species such as sheep or goats. Due to the strong bonds between donkeys and their owners, it is best to ask that person to catch and hold the donkey if they are capable. In addition, the strong bond between a donkey and its field companion means that it is important that, when handling a single animal, their bonded companion is present at the same time. Donkeys can become ill if they are separated from their companion, so it is important to keep companions together when handling.

Donkeys are very set in their routine, so it is best to perform any task within normal feeding or grooming time. If this is not possible, ask the owner to get the donkey used to be handled at different times of the day in the week leading up to the treatment required. As donkeys are wary of strangers it is important to give the donkey time to study you. Most donkeys are quite inquisitive and will, given time, come to investigate you.

As stoic species, donkeys do not display the usual signs of pain as other equids, but a small change in behaviour can be an indicator of pain. It is important whilst handling the donkey to pay close attention to behaviours such as kicking or trying to remove themselves from the situation. This behaviour could be due to pain and it is important to first eliminate this possibility before trying to correct the behaviour. Additionally, a donkey will behave according to its environment, and this includes the handler. If a handler is stressed or impatient, so will the donkey be! Make sure when handling or restraining the donkey that you remain calm and grounded.

8.1.3.3   How to Use Behavioural Traits to Effect when Handling Donkeys

A donkey that has an experienced, well-trained companion will be much easier to handle compared to a donkey that does not have this reassurance. By keeping companions together, any possible stress will be reduced. This will make handling much easier and will enable effective training to take place on how to behave when being caught and restrained. Well-handled donkeys are easy to catch and administer treatment to.

Donkeys are highly intelligent. It is important to give the donkey time to study a situation and to allow it to work things out. A donkey that does not want to perform a certain task will stand its ground. If a donkey does not want to do a task, the handler needs to work out why. Sheer force will encourage the donkey to stand its ground more and will not solve the problem. It must be remembered also that donkeys will give fewer overt signs about being aggressive. If a donkey is given time and a proper understanding of how it is to respond to situations, the easier a task will be to carry out and the better the experience is for all involved. As donkeys will stand still in a situation they are unsure of, it is possible to use this to your advantage when trying to catch a donkey in a small enough space. Follow the donkey into a corner, being careful not to stand directly behind it. Approaching calmly and gently, the handler should be able to place an arm over the donkeys' neck to catch it.

Donkeys tend to follow the general rule of where the head goes, the body goes. If you can get control of the head, handling and restraining should be much easier.

8.2   How to Approach a Horse/Donkey

The way in which you approach a horse or donkey will initially be determined by whether it is in a stable, small yard/paddock or a large field. You will then need to consider its temperament/behaviour and, if in a field, the number in the group and also the dynamics and social interaction within the group. As with farm animal species, horses and donkeys have a flight zone and, due to the position of the eyes, they have a blind spot directly behind them and directly beneath the muzzle. It is, therefore, always best to approach at the shoulder, which, as with other farm species, is their point of balance.

Approach the horse or donkey, preferably from the left side, with patience and with a quiet and calm demeanour. Use a calm tone of voice to make sure that it knows where you are at all times. Try to avoid directly making contact with the eyes and move towards it with the shoulders slightly turned away and the head down. When you are close, reaching out your hand with the palm facing down and allowing it to investigate you is good practice, particularly if it does not know you. If approaching with a lead rope and head collar, make sure that these are in the opposite hand and held either by the side or behind the back so they are not obvious.

Once you have approached its side, reach over the neck with your right arm and place the left hand on the dorsal aspect of the nose (unless of course height of the individual prevents this). This should bring it to a halt. Giving it a scratch on the withers as a reward for standing still is good practice and a good way to form a bond.

8.3   How to Put on a Head Collar and Lead in Hand

8.3.1   How to Put a Head Collar on a Horse in the Stable

Ensure that you check that the environment is safe before you enter the stable. Never put a head collar on over the stable door. On entering the stable close the door behind you and, as long as the horse is calm, secure the top bolt/latch. Should you feel that you may need a quick exit, then simply pull the door closed but do not lock it. If you are dealing with a difficult horse, you may need a second person to stand at the door to ensure that you can get out but the horse cannot. Approach the horse quietly from the left hand (near) side and stand at the horses shoulder, facing forward. Talking quietly can help reassure the horse and, once at the shoulder, placing a hand on the neck/withers will further aid reassurance. Never allow yourself to become trapped between the wall and the horse. Always try to get the horse to come over to you, wherever possible. Horses are inquisitive by nature and some positive reinforcement with a small treat will further aid this.

1) Place the end of the lead rope over the horse's neck. This will ensure that should the horse walk off; you will still have some control of the horse (Figure 8.3).
2) Carefully slip the noseband of the headcollar over the horse's muzzle and guide the noseband onto the bony part of the horse's head; this is roughly midpoint between the muzzle and the eyes (Figure 8.4).
   Make sure that you remain at the side of the horse and ensure that you are not either directly in front of the horse's head or front legs.
3) Place the headpiece of the head collar underneath the horse's neck and then over the poll (situated just behind the ears). Some horses can be head-shy around the ears, so take care when you are doing this. If the horse is head-shy, you may need to place the headpiece of the head collar much further back from the poll and slightly down the crest (Figure 8.5).
4) Fasten the head collar. You can now take the lead rope from the horse's neck and hold the lead rope in your left hand, with your right hand near the horse's chin (Figure 8.6).

Ensure that the head collar fits properly – this is important for safe restraint of the horse and also to ensure that the head collar is comfortable for the horse to wear. The noseband should sit approximately 2–3 fingers below the cheek bones of the horse and you should be able to comfortably fit two fingers between the nose of the horse and the noseband

You are now ready to either lead the horse out of the stable or tie the horse up using a quick release knot.

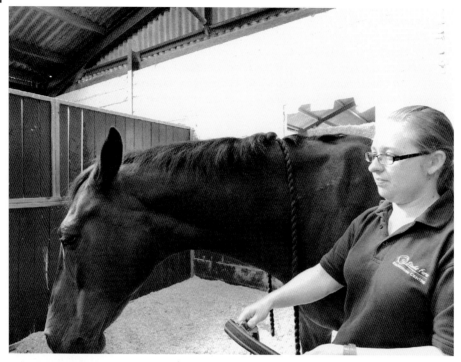

Figure 8.3 Putting on a head collar, Step 1 (Source: Courtesy of Brinsbury Campus, Chichester College).

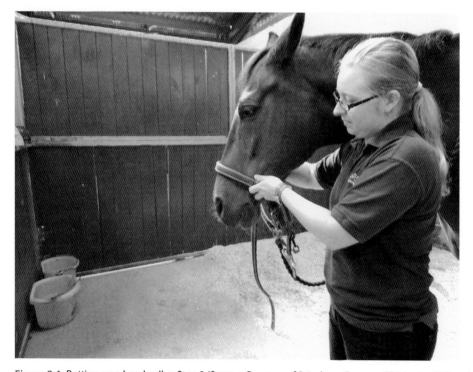

Figure 8.4 Putting on a head collar, Step 2 (Source: Courtesy of Brinsbury Campus, Chichester College).

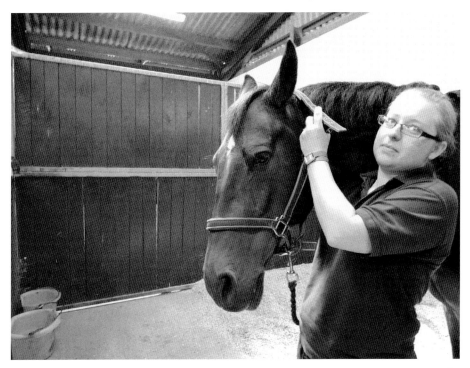

Figure 8.5 Putting on a head collar, Step 3 (Source: Courtesy of Brinsbury Campus, Chichester College).

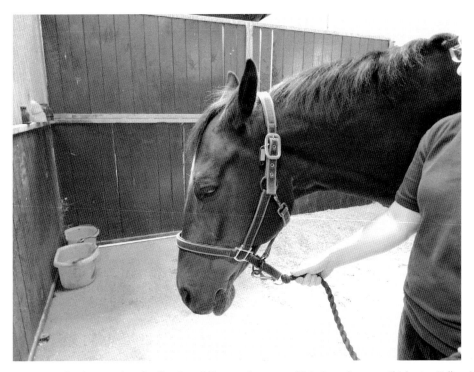

Figure 8.6 Putting on a head collar, Step 4 (Source: Courtesy of Brinsbury Campus, Chichester College).

8.3.2 How to Put a Head Collar on a Donkey in the Field

The procedure is much the same as that described for the horse above. When haltering a donkey, place the lead rope over the donkeys' neck so that it is out of the way whilst maintaining the hand on the front of the nose.

The rope over the neck also acts as a method of restraining the donkey if it were to move and get away from the handler (Figures 8.7 and 8.8).

Use both hands to place the nose strap of the halter over the donkeys' nose (Figure 8.9).

The left hand should hold the nose strap in place whilst the right hand should reach over the top of the donkeys' neck and pull the head strap up and over the back of the head of the donkey so that it reaches the fastening. Move the left hand at the same time sliding up the strap on the left side of the donkey where the fastening is (Figures 8.10 and 8.11).

Once the halter has been fastened using both hands, the right hand can be moved to hold the lead rope under the donkeys' chin and the left hand can hold the remaining section of the rope (Figure 8.12).

8.3.3 Quick Release Knot

There are a number of ways to tie a horse or donkey up using a quick release knot. The main thing to remember is that, whichever method you use, the lead rope must be placed

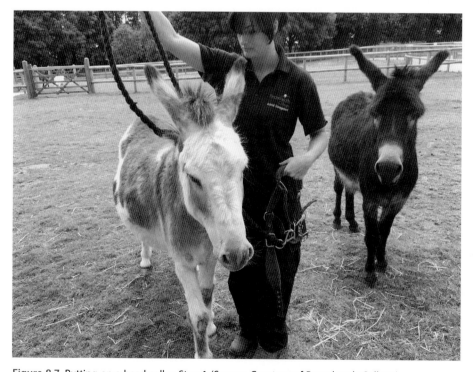

Figure 8.7 Putting on a head collar, Step 1 (Source: Courtesy of Reaseheath College).

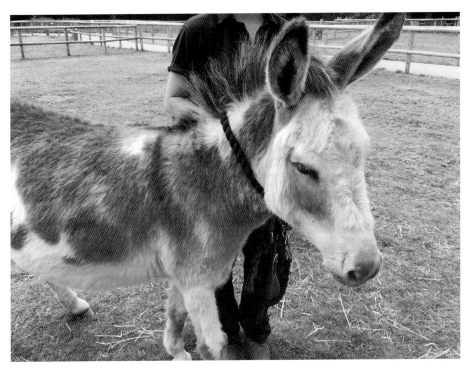

Figure 8.8 Putting on a head collar, Step 1 (Source: Courtesy of Reaseheath College).

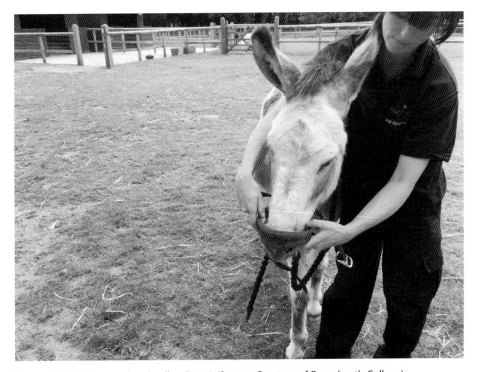

Figure 8.9 Putting on a head collar, Step 2 (Source: Courtesy of Reaseheath College).

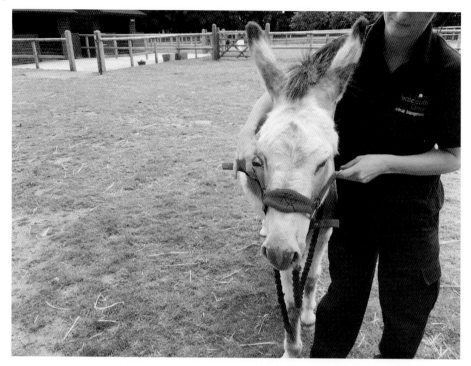

Figure 8.10 Putting on a head collar, Step 3 (Source: Courtesy of Reaseheath College).

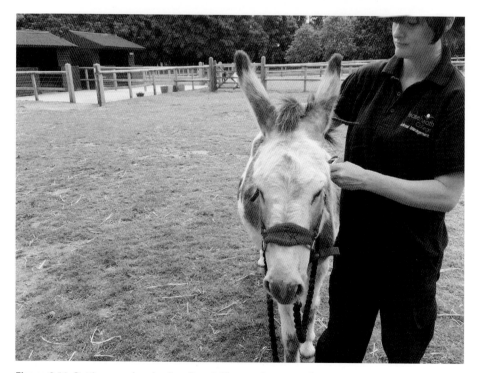

Figure 8.11 Putting on a head collar, Step 3 (Source: Courtesy of Reaseheath College).

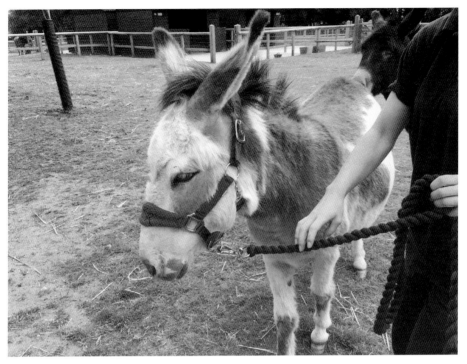

Figure 8.12 Putting on a head collar, Step 4 (Source: Courtesy of Reaseheath College).

through either a piece of baler twine or one of the new plastic snappers that have been designed for this purpose. An example method is described here.

1) Feed the lead rope from right to left through the baler twine (Figure 8.13).
2) Using the free end of the lead rope, make a circle by passing the free end over the end of the lead rope attached to the head collar (Figure 8.14).
3) Form the free end into a loop and pass this through the circle. Pull through the circle and tighten as you pull to form the quick release knot (Figures 8.15 and 8.16).

   DO NOT pass the free end of the rope through the formed loop. By doing this the knot will no longer be quick release.

8.3.4   How to Lead in Hand

Holding the lead rope correctly with the right hand under the animals chin and the left hand holding the remaining rope, the animal should be asked to walk forward with a little pull of the rope under the chin and a voice command. Most horses and donkeys will happily be led to an area they are familiar with. If they are not sure about the surroundings or what they are being asked to do, they may resist moving forward. Give them time to work out what is being asked of them, then ask again in the same manner. If pressure is applied at both the front and from behind, the pressure from behind can be a distraction. Try to only lead and encourage them forward from the front or the side. If they are being moved with a companion this can make it easier, especially if

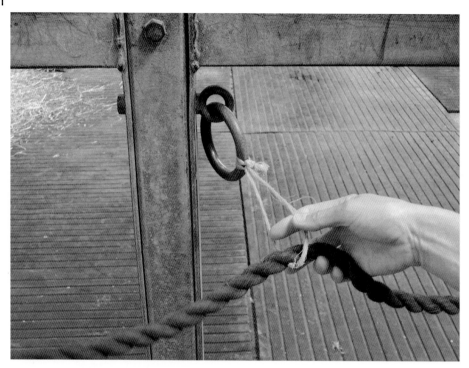

Figure 8.13 Quick release knot, Step 1.

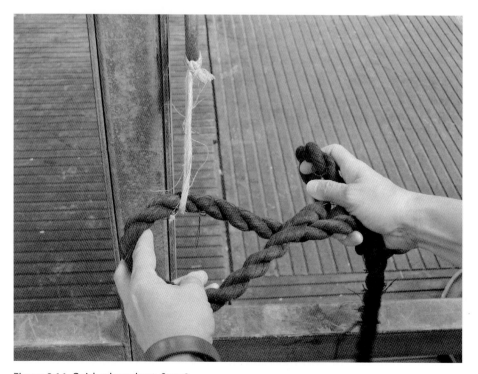

Figure 8.14 Quick release knot, Step 2.

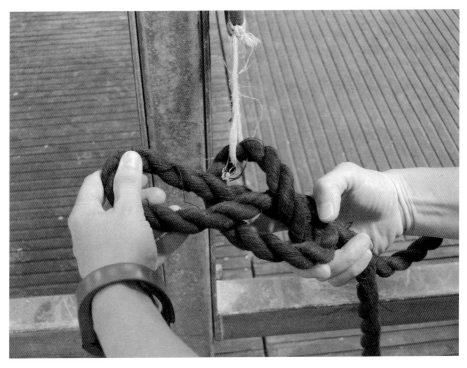

Figure 8.15 Quick release knot, Step 3.

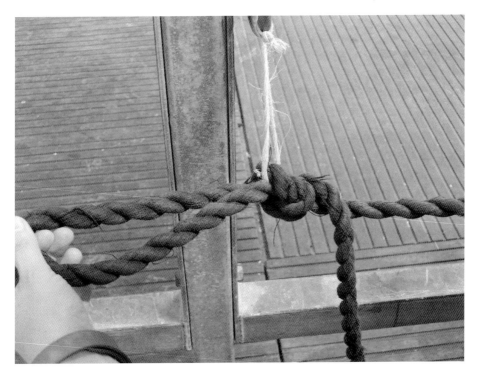

Figure 8.16 Quick release knot, Step 3.

Table 8.2 General principles of restraint (Loving and Johnston, 1995).

Principle	Description
Environment	Working in a familiar environment will make the horse feel secure; if necessary ensure that the horse's normal companions are nearby; try to ensure that the yard/stable environment is quiet.
Reassurance	Take the time to reassure the horse and use positive reinforcement (i.e. food treats); do not hurry with the procedure and take time to gain the trust of the horse.
Confidence and patience	Humans easily transmit fear and nervousness, so it is important that acts are decisive and not hesitant; slow and deliberate movements will build confidence; above all, remain calm and do not lose your temper.
Psychology	A horse should always be reacting to the people and not the other way round; in other words you will need to be one step ahead of the horse and try to anticipate what the horse will do; this method of training requires empathy; restraint is not about physical force.

the companion is more experienced. Horses and donkeys will also respond to treats such as a biscuit or carrot.

Never wrap the lead rope around your hand.

8.4 Physical Restraint

Whenever restraining a horse or donkey, care must be taken to observe its behaviour for the subtle signs of stress or pain. It must be remembered that just because it does not respond, does not mean that it is not experiencing stress or pain.

The degree and type of restraint required will depend on the individual animals' temperament, age and previous handling experience. Wherever possible, try to use the minimal amount of restraint required by each animal to reduce stress and also to try to minimize the risk of unwanted behaviours that can occur due to a bad experience with handling. There are some general principles that can be applied to the restraint of any horse (Table 8.2).

8.5 Methods and Equipment

8.5.1 Head Collar

Head collars and halters are the simplest means by which you can restrain a horse or donkey. Whenever you are working with or around an individual, it should always be wearing a head collar to afford you some means of restraint. You should never work around an animal with no means by which to restrain it. Head collars come in a variety of sizes, so it is important that you select the correct size in order to ensure the comfort of the individual and also to ensure that the head collar works on the correct pressure point (i.e. the bridge of the nose). Rope halters can also be used; however, you need to ensure that these are put on correctly and are secure. If they are too tight and left in place for too long, they can cause damage to the sensitive parts of the head.

8.5.2 Bridle

There are many different types of bridles that are used for riding horses and the choice of bridle will very much depend on the individual horse and what it is being used for. When handling a horse from the ground a bridle is often used for restraint when more control is required, for example when the horse is being trotted up for examination. It is important that the simplest form of bit is used in order to ensure that the pressure of the bit in the mouth does not cause pain to the horse. As with the head collar, it is important that the bridle is fitted correctly (Figure 8.17, 8.18 and 8.19).

8.5.3 Chiffney Bit

The chiffney bit (also known as the anit-rearing bit) is designed to be used for horses that are difficult to handle or, more specifically, for handling stallions. It was invented by Samuel Chiffney Senior (a racing jockey) and patented in 1805. It is particularly popular for use in the horseracing industry and the British Horseracing Authority (BHA) rules that 'you have to use a bridle or a head collar fitted with a Chiffney when a horse is being led on site at a racecourse' (BHA, ND).

It is not a bit that is used for riding horses. Its use is also somewhat controversial, as if used incorrectly it can do a lot of damage to the horse's mouth and cause considerable pain. The mouthpiece, which applies pressure to the tongue and the bars of the mouth, is a thin metal circle that loops over the horse's tongue and behind the chin and is attached to a single-strap headpiece. The lead rope attaches to a single loose ring at the back of the horse's chin (Figures 8.20 and 8.21). It is best to be used in conjunction with a head collar.

8.5.4 Twitch

The use of the twitch has received attention in recent years due to its potential to be misused, despite it being a method of restraint that is commonly used in equine yards. The principle behind the use of the twitch is that it applies pressure to an area of the horse's skin that, as previously mentioned, has sensory nerves and acts by causing the release of endorphins from the central nervous system, thereby causing the horse to relax. The twitch should only be used for short procedures.

It also acts as a distractor, thereby allowing a procedure to be performed, for example a neck twitch (Figure 8.22) can be applied to the horse at the same time as giving a vaccination.

The controversy around the use of the twitch is with regards to the fact that when applied to certain areas of the horses body, such as the ear (Figure 8.23) and upper lip (Figure 8.24), a degree of pain is to be expected and it is the pain of application that horses are responding to. When used incorrectly, the twitch can also be associated with learned and aversive behaviours, that is the horse that becomes head-shy following the application of an ear twitch. It is recommended that ear twitching is not carried out on any horse or donkey.

Figure 8.25 shows a home-made rope twitch; this is the most common type of nose twitch found in equine yards. The handle in this image is really too long and should be shorter. Also, it would be better if the handle was made of polypipe rather than wood,

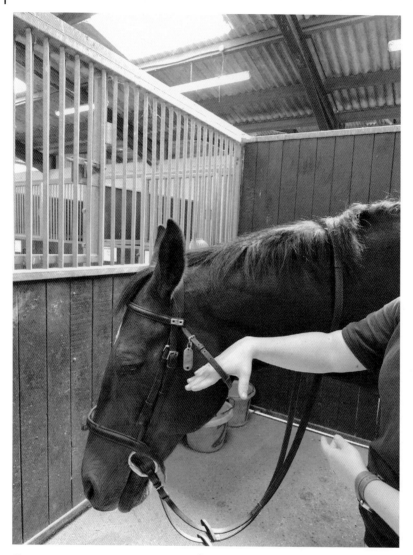

Figure 8.17 Correct fitting of the throat latch (one hand width) on the bridle (Source: Courtesy of Brinsbury Campus, Chichester College).

as if a horse were to fling his head in the air, there is a real risk of the twitch hitting the handler in the head. It is important as well to ensure that the rope or twine used for the loop is as soft and wide as possible to prevent damage to the sensitive skin of the upper lip.

Figures 8.26 and 8.27 show a humane twitch, which, as the name suggests, is supposed to be better for the horse's welfare. However, these are not widely used, as they tend to not be as effective as the more common rope twitch. They are, nevertheless, recommended for use and are preferable for inexperienced handlers.

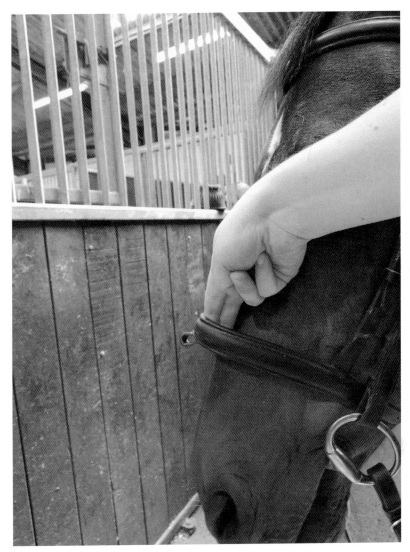

Figure 8.18 Correctly fitting snaffle bridle with cavesson noseband (Source: Courtesy of Brinsbury Campus, Chichester College).

How to correctly apply a twitch to a horse is shown in Figure 8.28.

Step 1 – It is easier if the person who is applying the twitch holds the horse. It is also preferable that the handler wears a hard hat, especially when applying a twitch to a horse whose behaviour is unknown. With the lead rope over your shoulder, place one hand on the lead rope and with your left hand place your fingers through the rope loop (Figure 8.28).

Steps 2 and 3 – Using the fingers of your left hand, gently take hold of the horses' upper lip and slide the rope over your fingers and up over the upper lip (Figure 8.29). This is a good point to gauge the reaction of the horse and whether it is safe to proceed.

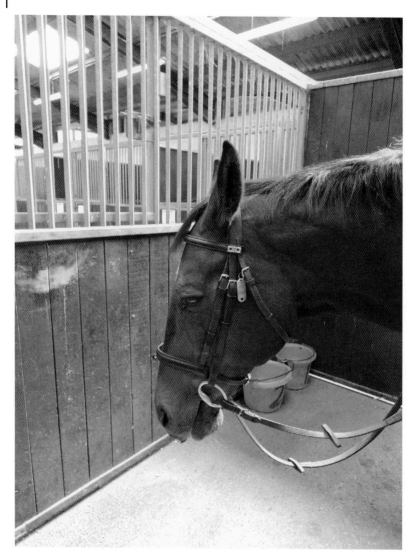

Figure 8.19 Correctly fitting snaffle bridle with cavesson noseband (Source: Courtesy of Brinsbury Campus, Chichester College).

If it is safe to continue, twist the handle of the twitch in a clockwise direction to tighten the loop around the upper lip (Figure 8.30). Note that some horses that have very sensitive muzzles may at this time try to wriggle the loop off. Do not overtighten the loop.

8.5.5 Stocks

Stocks allow for a horse to be completely confined in an enclosed area and severely limits its movements. However, horses may still bite and kick even with this method of restraint. There are many designs of stocks for equine use and the type employed will

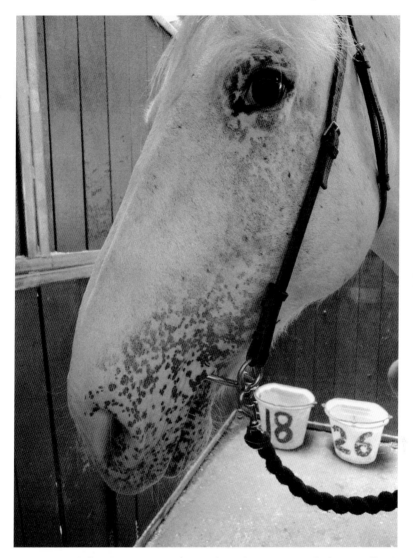

Figure 8.20 Chiffney bit (Source: Courtesy of Brinsbury Campus, Chichester College).

depend on its use. For the majority of equine yards, this is an expensive piece of equipment and, therefore, not a justified expense. The main places you will find these being used are in breeding establishments and veterinary hospitals.

8.5.6 Tail Restraint

With some procedures, such as picking up a hind foot, it may be beneficial to hold the horses' tail to provide some further restraint. In order to kick the horse will generally clamp the tail between the back legs. Whenever moving around the horse it is important to stay as close to the horse as possible and maintain light pressure on the body. This way,

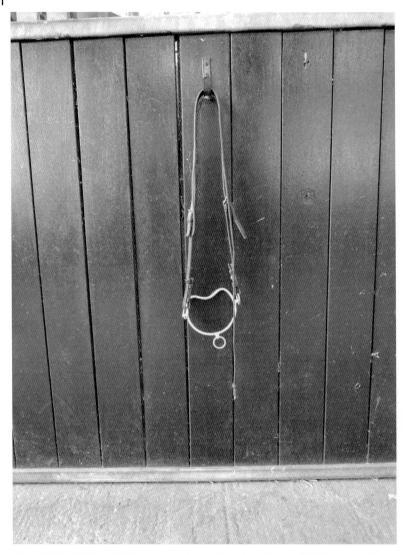

Figure 8.21 Chiffney bit (Source: Courtesy of Brinsbury Campus, Chichester College).

the handler is able to feel whether a horse is becoming tense, and also if the horse does kick the force of the impact will be less. Figures 8.31, 8.32, 8.33 and 34 show how to correctly restrain the tail.

Step 1 – Moving from the horses withers and staying close to the horse, place the hand closest to the tail on the hindquarters.

Step 2 – Place your hand around the top of the tail.

Step 3 – Gently pull the tail towards you.

Step 4 – Move the hand down the tail until you are in a comfortable position and feel a slight pull of the horse towards you.

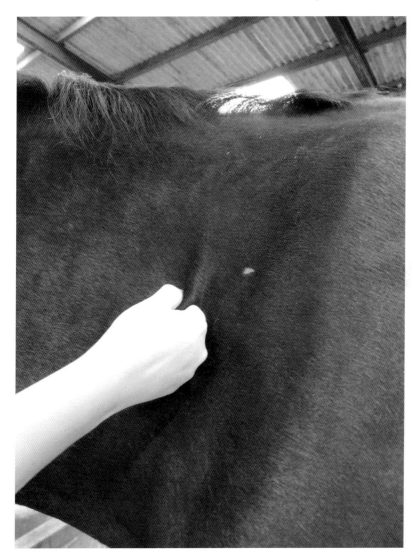

Figure 8.22 Neck twitch (Source: Courtesy of Brinsbury Campus, Chichester College).

8.5.7 Physical Restraint of Donkeys

A well-handled donkey should easily be restrained through the use of a halter, which can either be held by an assistant or can be tied using a quick release knot to thin twine. Once the donkey cannot get away by pulling its handler, it is likely to remain still. An extra hand under the chin by the handler can help to prevent the donkey from moving forward and away from the handler.

If the donkey will not stand still using just a halter, a donkey bridle can be used to get better control of the head. If using a bridle for extra restraint an assistant must be present to hold the donkey. The donkey must not be tied with a bridle.

If the donkey will still not stand still, further restraint can be applied by holding up a front leg (Figure 8.35). The handler should stand by the shoulder facing the hindquarters

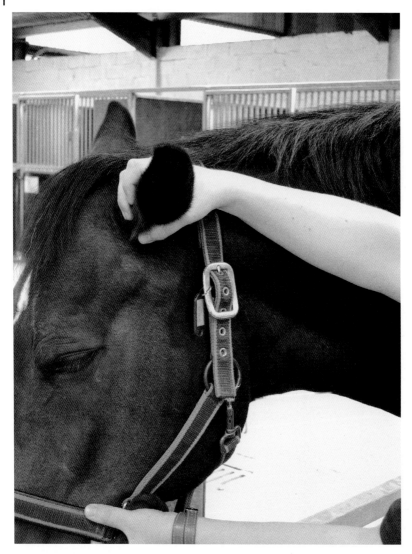

Figure 8.23 Ear twitch (Source: Courtesy of Brinsbury Campus, Chichester College).

of the donkey and lift a front leg up by running the closest hand down the back of the leg and upon reaching the foot, giving a command and gently pull to encourage the donkey to lift the leg themselves. The leg must be held in a position that is comfortable for the donkey and the handler. However, lifting of a front leg can be unreliable as donkeys have a good ability to stand on two legs and still carefully place a kick.

Further restraint can be applied through the use of a blindfold. This can be as simple as cupping a hand over the donkeys' eye near to the handler or where the treatment is taking place. The use of a twitch is not effective on donkeys as it does not have the same effect on donkeys as it does in other equids. However, an ear can be gently grasped at the base and held (Figure 8.36) gently squeezing the sides together. The ear must never be twisted or pulled.

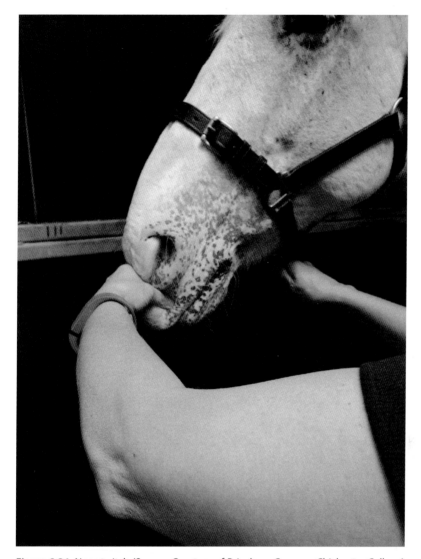

Figure 8.24 Nose twitch (Source: Courtesy of Brinsbury Campus, Chichester College).

8.6 Training for Restraint

To be able to train a horse, it is important to understand how a horse learns and, in order to do this, it is necessary to have a basic understanding of the 'theory of learning'. Part of the learning process stems from memory and whilst horses have an excellent long-term memory (Wolff and Hausberger, 1996) they have a poor short-term memory. Much of how they learn is through trial and error and a process of operant conditioning, classical conditioning and habituation (Pearson, 2015).

Habituation is considered to be the simplest form of learning and is the long-term, stimulus-specific waning of a response, for example a horse habituates to the feel of a

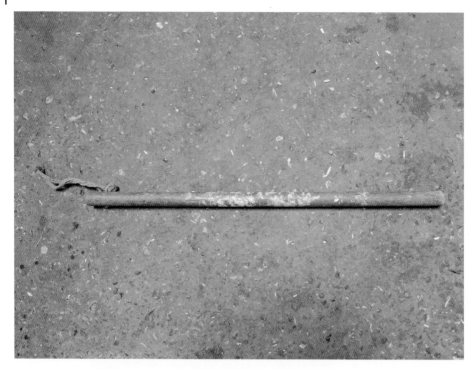

Figure 8.25 Rope twitch.

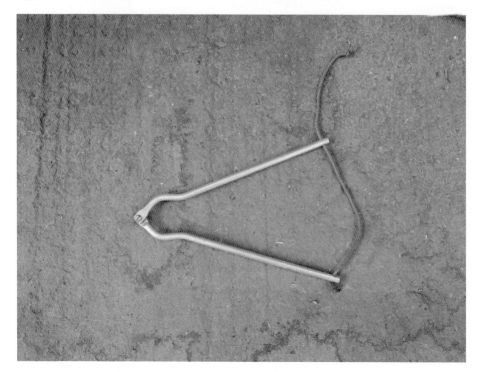

Figure 8.26 Humane twitch.

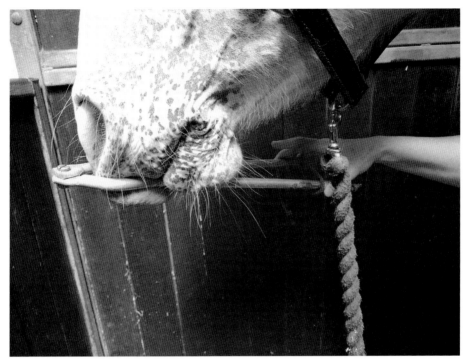

Figure 8.27 Humane twitch loosely applied (Source: Courtesy of Brinsbury Campus, Chichester College).

head collar on its head. Many of the techniques used to restrain a horse are accomplished via habituation.

Many handlers will also use forms of positive and negative reinforcement in order to shape a horses behaviour. In its simplest form, positive reinforcement would be to offer a food treat when a positive response to a task is offered. However, in the equine world, negative reinforcement is perhaps one of the main ways in which we train horses. For example, if you keep pulling on the horse's mouth with the bit, the horse will eventually stop pulling as it will want to evade the pain that is caused. One does need to be careful though not to confuse negative reinforcement with punishment. For example, the use of the whip if a horse refuses a jump. Here it is timing of the whip that is most important, as the horse must associate the punishment with refusing to jump.

It is important to stress that, on welfare grounds, positive reinforcement should always be used whenever possible.

8.6.1 Training Donkeys for Restraint

Donkeys (and their hybrids) are highly intelligent and respond well to training. It must be remembered that donkeys are very sensitive to their environments and this includes the handler. If a handler is nervous for example, the donkey will pick up on this and become nervous of the situation it finds itself in. Before commencing any training, the handler

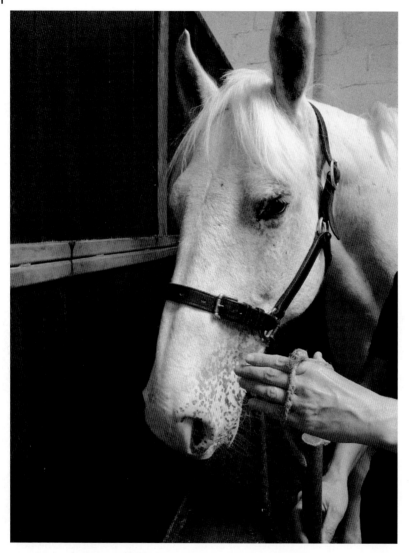

Figure 8.28 Applying a twitch, Step 1 (Source: Courtesy of Brinsbury Campus, Chichester College).

must have a good understanding of donkey behaviour, particularly with regards reading the subtle signals of a donkey's body language. Getting to know an individual well and how that individual donkey learns, is key to successful training.

The creation of a safe environment to work in and a training plan are also key steps to effective training. Donkeys must not be rushed and small steps at a time should be taken. Make sure to reward any good behaviour but to ignore any unwanted or bad behaviour. Donkeys must be given time to work out what is being asked of them. If the handler/ trainer is impatient or unclear in what they are asking of the donkey, this will slow the learning process down. Procedures such as lifting of the foot are very unnatural to the

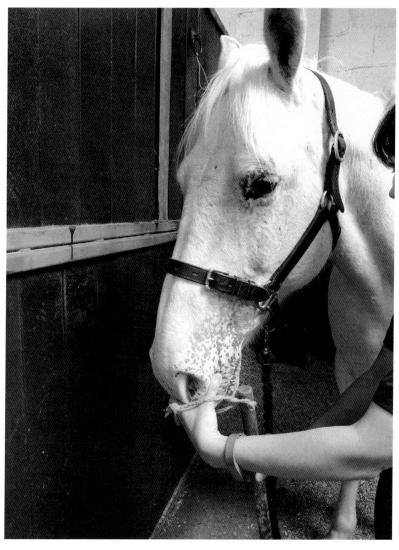

Figure 8.29 Applying a twitch, Steps 2 and 3 (Source: Courtesy of Brinsbury Campus, Chichester College).

donkey, so will take longer to learn than something that is closer to its more natural behaviour. Thus, it is important to make sure that you are only asking it to perform one behaviour at a time.

Donkeys will quickly learn to avoid any activity that is either difficult or painful, or that they have not been given enough time to process. A donkey will quickly come to fear anybody that has been involved in a situation that induced pain or fear. Well-handled donkeys will be motivated to learn new things and are easier to train. Good communication and patience from the handler are key to a successful training experience.

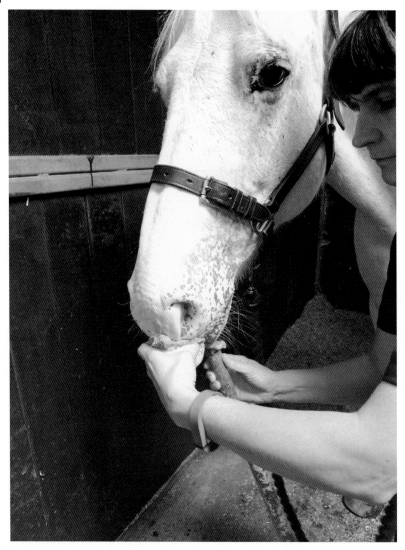

Figure 8.30 Applying a twitch, Steps 2 and 3 (Source: Courtesy of Brinsbury Campus, Chichester College).

8.7 Handling and Restraint of Foals

8.7.1 Development of Behaviour

There are many time points that define the behavioural development of foals. Within the first hour of life, the foal will be able to stand and move towards its mother in an attempt to suckle. The foal will also be stimulated by its mother licking it to respond to auditory and visual stimuli, and thus begin to communicate with 'nickers' to its mother and by snapping at any fearful object. Within the first day of life the foal is able to play, urinate,

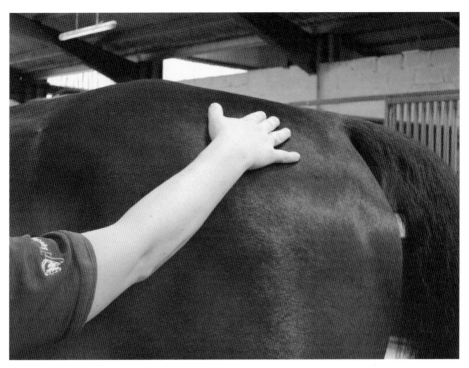

Figure 8.31 Tail restraint, Step 1 (Source: Courtesy of Brinsbury Campus, Chichester College).

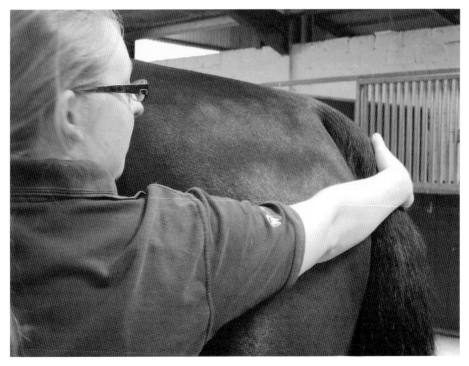

Figure 8.32 Tail restraint, Step 2 (Source: Courtesy of Brinsbury Campus, Chichester College).

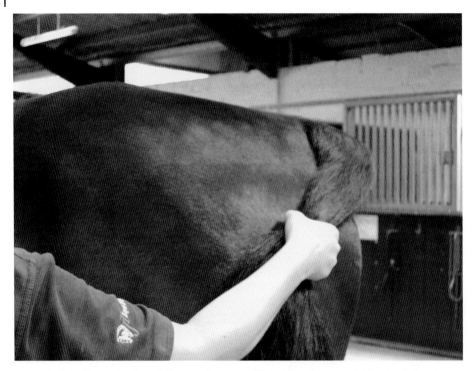

Figure 8.33 Tail restraint, Step 3 (Source: Courtesy of Brinsbury Campus, Chichester College).

flehmen and graze, as well as communicate (Houpt, 2011). The mare–foal bond starts to develop as soon as the foal is born and the amount of distance between the mare and foal is proportional to the age of the foal, that is the younger the foal, the closer it stays to the mare.

When working with foals it is important to be aware that you as a handler will have a direct effect on shaping behaviour at an important stage when the foal will be learning. Handling of foals requires calm and patience, as, whilst you may be able to manhandle them when they are very young, they will quickly grow and any negative handling experiences will be more difficult to deal with in an adult horse. There are many horses that develop behavioural issues when they are young and being poorly handled is one of the contributory factors. Foals will also bond with human carers; this is seen, especially, in orphan foals that are hand-reared. Wherever possible it is preferable to have a surrogate mother rear a foal.

8.7.2 Restraint of Foals

Foals can be handled from birth as long as the handler does not interfere with the maternal bonding that is important between the mare and foal early in life. It is important, though, that the young foal is handled by humans from an early age in order that as it grows size does not become a barrier to safe restraint. Many foals habituate to wearing a head collar and being led in hand beside the mare from as early as a couple of days of age.

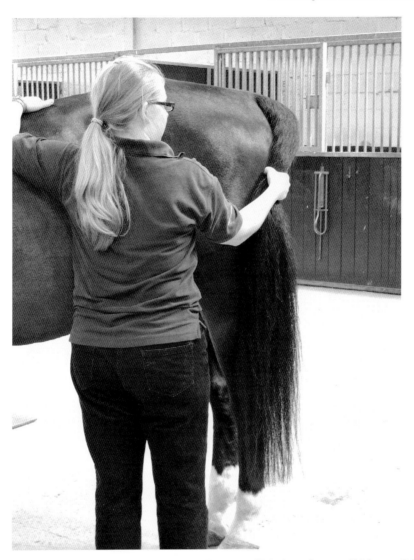

Figure 8.34 Tail restraint, Step 4 (Source: Courtesy of Brinsbury Campus, Chichester College).

When restraining a foal it is important not to place too much pressure on the head, as this can often lead to frustration and aversive behaviour by the foal. It is much better to simply encircle the foal with one arm placed around the chest and the other around behind the hindquarters. With an older or bigger foal, placing the foal against a wall and putting a knee firmly into the flank is usually enough to keep the foal still. It is important to be quiet and calm with foals, as they can move very quickly and will buck and rear in order to try to escape the handler. Also, be very mindful of the mare, as if mare's feels that its foal is being threatened it will become anxious and may even be aggressive towards the handler.

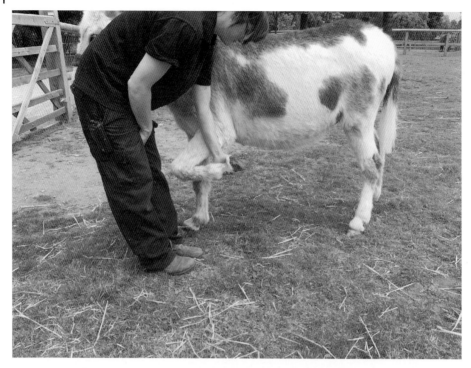

Figure 8.35 Picking up a front leg (Source: Courtesy of Reaseheath College).

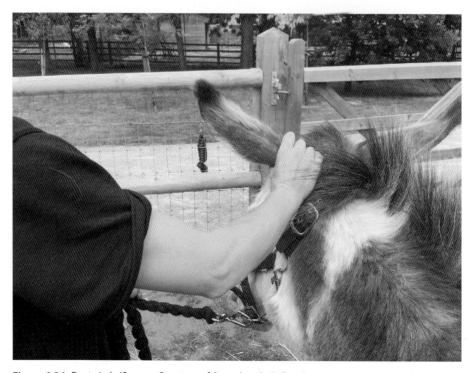

Figure 8.36 Ear twitch (Source: Courtesy of Reaseheath College).

8.8 Handling and Restraint of Stallions

Great care must always be taken with the handling and restraint of stallions and only experienced handlers should be given this responsibility, particularly if a stallion is being used for breeding and it is in the breeding season. The minimum restraint for any stallion would be a well-fitting bridle and stallions should never be restrained in a head collar alone. As with any horse, the temperament and behaviour of the individual stallion, age and also what the stallion is used for will impact on restraint methods employed. However, it is important to emphasize that a calm, confident manner around stallions is imperative. As with any horse, stallions will be able to sense nervousness and hesitancy in the handler and, whilst a firm hand is required with handling, this should not be confused with excessive force.

Key Points

- Whilst the majority of injuries to humans in their association with horses is caused due to riding accidents, 30–40% of injuries happen to people on the ground, near the horse.
- Many owners and trainers of horses will state that assessing a horse's temperament is important for breeding and performance. However, there is currently no recognized standard method available for temperament assessment.
- Donkeys do not express overt signs of pain or stress. They are much more subtle in their expression and this must be considered at all time.
- A donkey must be given time to work out what you as a handler are asking of it.
- You must cooperate with a donkey; sheer force will not bring about movement.
- Bonded donkeys should be kept together at all times, where possible.
- A twitch does not work on a donkey as it does on horses.
- A good understanding of the behaviour of horses and donkeys is key for effective training.
- It is important to stress that on welfare grounds positive reinforcement should always be used whenever possible.

Self-assessment Questions

1 How is handling of a donkey influenced by the fact that naturally they can live solitary lives?

2 With regards handling, what is the importance of the bond between a pair of donkeys?

3 How does placing a hand under the chin of the donkey prevent it from moving forward?

4 What are the dangers involved in holding a donkeys front leg for restraint?

5　Why should the twitch only be used for short procedures and where (anatomically) is it recommended not to twitch a horse?

6　How would you restrain a foal?

Answers can be found in the back of the book.

References

BHA (ND) Trainer Manual: The Rules of Racing, British Horseracing Authority (rules. britishhorseracing.com/pdf/BHA_rules_export_126042.pdf; last accessed 27 May 2017).

Cohen, J. (2012) Horse domestication happened across Eurasia, study shows. http://www.history.com/news/horse-domestication-happened-across-eurasia-study-shows; last accessed 27 May 2017.

Goodwin, D. (1999) The importance of ethology in understanding the behaviour of the horse. *Equine Veterinary Journal*, **31** (28 Suppl), 15–19.

Horsetalk (2007) World horse population estimated at 58 million. http://www.horsetalk.co.nz/2007/09/12/world-horse-population-58m/#axzz4H1pJC7vC; last accessed 27 May 2017.

Houpt, K.A. (2011) *Domestic Animal Behaviour for Veterinarians and Animal Scientists*, 5th edn, John Wiley & Sons Ltd, Chichester.

Kimura, B., Marshall, F., Beja-Pereira, A. and Mulligan, C. (2013) Donkey Domestication. *African Archaeological Review*, **30** (1), 83–95.

Loving, N.S. and Johnston, A.M. (1995) *Veterinary Manual for the Performance Horse*. Blackwell Science, Oxford.

McGreevy, P. (2004) Current research: equine behaviour. *Journal of Equine Veterinary Science*, **24** (9), 397–398.

Miller, R.M. (2006) Behaviour. In: *The Equine Manual*, 2nd edn (eds A.J. Higgins and J.R. Snyder), Elsevier Saunders: Edinburgh.

Moehlman, P.D., Kebede, F. and Yohannes, H. (2015) *Equus africanus*. The IUCN Red List of Threatened Species 2015. http://dx.doi.org/10.2305/IUCN.UK.2015-2.RLTS.T7949A45170994.en; last accessed 27 May 2017.

Murray, L.M.A., Byrne, K. and D'Eath, R.B. (2013). Pair-bonding and companion recognition in domestic donkeys *Equus asinus*. *Applied Animal Behaviour Science*, **143**, 67–74.

Pearson, G. (2015) Practical application of learning theory. *In Practice*, **37**, 251–254.

Proops, L., Burden, F. and Osthaus, B. (2012) Social relations in a mixed group of mules, ponies and donkeys reflect differences in equid type. *Behavioural Processes*, **90**, 337–342.

Riley, C.B., Liddiard, J.R. and Thompson, K. (2015) A cross-sectional study of horse-related injuries in veterinary and animal science students at an Australian university. *Animals*, **5**, 951–964. doi: 10.3390/ani5040392.

Rossel, S., Marshall, F., Peters, J. *et al.* (2008) Domestication of the donkey: timing, processes and indicators. *Proceedings of the National Academy of Sciences*, **105** (10), 3715–3720.

Sorli, J.M. (2000) Equestrian injuries: a five year review of hospital admissions in British Columbia, *Canada. Injury Prevention*, **6**, 59–61.

Starkey, P. and Starkey, M. (1998) Regional and world trends in donkey populations. www.atnesa.org/donkeys/donkeys-starkey-populations.pdf; last accessed 27 May 2017.

Wolff, A. and Hausberger, M. (1996) Learning and memorisation of two different tasks in horses: the effects of age, sex and sire. *Applied Animal Behaviour Science*, **44**, 137–143.

Further Reading

Osthaus, B., Proops, L., Hocking, I. and Burden, F. (2013) Spatial cognition and perseveration by horses, donkeys and mules in simple A-not-B detour task. *Animal Cognition*, **16**, 301–305.

Proops, L., Burden, F. and Osthaus, B. (2009) Mule cognition: a case of hybrid vigour? *Animal Cognition*, **12**, 75–84.

9

Handling and Restraint of Cattle

Krista M. McLennan[1] and Stella J. Chapman[2]

[1]*Chester University, Chester, UK*
[2]*University Centre Hartpury, Gloucestershire, UK*

The timeline for the domestication of cattle is not as straight forward as for other species, such as the dog, and there have been many conflicting studies over the years that have tried to trace the history of their domestication. It is not until recently, with the aid of mitochondrial DNA analysis, that more accurate details of domestication have unfolded.

Modern cattle breeds are descended from multiple independent domestication events that occurred approximately 10 000 years ago (McTavish *et al.*, 2013). Wild cattle or aurochs (*Bos primigenius*) were most likely domesticated independently on two or three separate occasions and the cave paintings of Lascaux (France) depict archaeological evidence of the aurochs from the Upper Paleolithic hunters of Europe. Archaeological and biological evidence indicate that domestication events were geographical in nature, with *Bos taurus* in the near east and *Bos indicus* in the Indus valley of the Indian subcontinent. More recent mitochondrial DNA research indicates *Bos taurus* were introduced into Europe and Africa, where they interbred with aurochs. American descendants of cattle are thought to have been introduced in the late 1400s by explorers to the New World and were of *Bos taurus* lineage (McTavish *et al.*, 2013).

It is important to note that modern cattle are significantly different from the first domesticates.

9.1 Behaviour

9.1.1 Dairy and Beef Cattle

Cattle are a prey species and will see their handler as a potential threat until they have learnt otherwise. In a threatening situation, cattle's main line of defence is to try and remove themselves. If they cannot do this, then they are likely to rely on their speed, body, head and hooves. This can lead them to pushing the handler against a fence, into other animals or charging through you. Animals that have horns can lead to gorging; nevertheless, even polled animals can cause serious injury. Cattle should be respected for their strength and natural prey behaviour, and must be handled in a considerate and humane manner.

Cattle are naturally very sociable and have a strong herding instinct. Cattle herds have a natural hierarchy with subordinate and dominant individuals, as well as leaders and followers. Cattle that are separated away from other herd members will become increasingly anxious and frightened and thus dangerous.

Cattle have a very keen sense of hearing and vision. The eyes of cattle are on the sides of their head giving them almost 360° vision around their bodies, with a small blind spot directly behind them. Cattle have primarily monocular vision, which limits their ability to judge the size and speed of objects that are approaching. They are only able to judge this in a small area at the front of their nose where their vision becomes binocular. Cattle are dichromate's, meaning that they do not have the ability to see red. They are more likely to see in varying shades of browns and greys.

Cattle are naturally curious as a prey animal, showing interest in new people or objects within their environments. However, novelty can increase the arousal level of cattle and, subsequently, increase the level of excitability or fear. Highly aroused cattle can be difficult to handle and should be given time to settle before any handling is carried out.

The behaviour of beef and dairy cattle will differ due to the different rearing and management systems employed. Fewer problems occur when handling dairy cattle compared to beef, as dairy cattle will have experienced more regular, predictable handling than beef cattle. Beef cattle also rear their young until time of weaning, increasing the protective behaviours displayed by beef cows. In comparison, dairy calves are reared away from mothers in smaller groups with regular contact with humans. Individuals will also vary in temperament. This can differ between and within breeds, and individuals reared together in the same group will differ in temperament. Individual temperaments should be identified during history taking and before any handling commences.

9.2 How to Use Behavioural Traits to Good Effect When Handling

9.2.1 Cattle as a Prey Animal

Good handling gets a job done quickly, safely and efficiently. Cattle can be easily spooked by sudden movement and panicked cattle can be very dangerous and often slip and cause themselves injury. If cattle cannot escape from a situation that they do not feel comfortable with, they will often freeze and potentially go down. 'Downer cattle' should be given time to stand in their own time. This may take several minutes and they may stand suddenly. If they cannot return to their feet unaided, help should be provided in the form of a mechanical device such a cattle hoist.

When carrying out any handling with cattle, it is important that their perception of the environment is considered. They have a keen sense of smell and very good hearing, so any strong smells or noises can be highly distracting. Whenever handling cattle, avoid loud noises such as yelling, isolation and distractions. Due to their ability to only see varying shades of green and brown, they are more prone to seeing striking differences between light and dark, which can cause them to balk. It is important to be aware of this, especially when moving between the inside and outside of buildings.

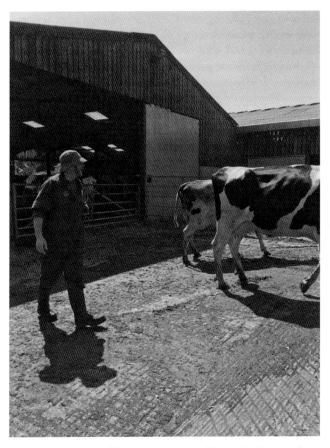

Figure 9.1 Using the flight zone to move dairy cattle (Source: Courtesy of Reaseheath College).

9.2.2 Flight Zone and Point of Balance

Understanding the 'flight zone' and 'point of balance' principles are key to stress-free handling of cattle. The flight zone is an area of personal space around the individual or group of cattle. When a handler enters this space the cattle will move away from the handler, re-establishing their personal space. The direction in which cattle move will depend on the angle of the handler to the shoulder or 'point of balance' (Figure 9.1). Working at a 45–60° angle behind the shoulder will move the cow forward. Moving back and forth parallel to the direction you want the animal to move will encourage the animal to walk in the desired direction. It is important that the handler works on the edge of the flight zone in a calm and considerate manner in order to avoid the animal balking, rearing or running away. Individual cattle will have their own flight zone and this will vary with temperament, arousal level and previous experience of being handled. Note that the flight zone is larger near to the head than it is to the tail end of the cow. This is due to their eyesight and range of vision, with a blind spot directly behind the tail.

9.2.3 Cattle as a Social Species

Cattle must be moved as a group. You must be patient and use deliberate and slow movements. If cattle break off from the main herd, sit and wait for them to return to the main group before continuing on. This will be quicker and more effective compared to chasing them. Making use of a leader of the group by encouraging the leader to come to you, bringing all the cows with her rather than having to go and collect the cows, is the most stress-free method for all concerned, but it can take time to build the relationship to this level and groups must be stable in their make-up. A group leader is likely to be a middle ranking cow. Dominant cattle tend to walk in the middle of a group with subordinate cattle at the back of the group, with the leaders up the front. This is why pushing a group from behind will not speed up the movement of the group. It is the leaders that will set the pace and subordinate cattle do not want to enter into the personal spaces of dominant individuals. Be aware of any cattle that are trailing behind the group, as they may be lame or unwell. Go as slow as the last cow.

When penning cattle, they should never be isolated from others. This is highly stressful. Where an individual needs to be handled, keep a small group of cattle close by so that the individual cow can see and hear them as a minimum. Being in contact with another animal will keep the cow calm, making handling safer and quicker. Mother cows can be very protective of their calves, and bulls of their cows. Where possible separate adult cattle away from youngsters and bulls away from cows and calves. It is easier to separate calm cattle away from highly aroused cattle, leaving the aroused cattle in the pen. Before carrying out any handling after cattle have been collected, ideally they should be left to settle. This should be about 20–30 minutes. As there is a natural hierarchy in a group, it is important that you do not overcrowd the area. Subordinate animals that are in close confinement with dominant animals without means of escape will be susceptible to injury, as they will not be able to avoid the dominant individuals. Cattle should be afforded room to move away freely from others in order to prevent behavioural problems, such cattle becoming highly aroused, or excessive aggression taking place.

9.2.4 Previous Experience

Previous handling experienced by cattle can have a dramatic effect on their reaction the next time around. Cattle that experience positive relationships with their handlers on a regular basis from early on in life are calmer and easier to handle. Positive handling can also allow a handler to calm a cow that may be anxious during a procedure. The gentle placing of a hand on a cow can be very effective if they are anxious or unsettled. Cattle that are not used to being handled or have only experienced negative handling before, can have a high level of arousal, making them particularly dangerous to work with. Dairy cattle tend to have a fairly strict routine and may well be waiting at a gate to come in for milking or food. This can be made use of by encouraging the cows to come to you at this time with a positive reward such as food. Be careful, however, that any changes to their routine are slow, as it can impact on the milk yield of dairy cattle. This can also impact on how they perceive the handling process, so timing of handling should be considered. Cattle tend to be easier to handle after milking and after they have been fed.

Cattle have good memories and will respond well to early gentle handling. Cattle that have been exposed to gentle handing since they were calves will be much easier to handle than cattle that were not. Encouraging stockpersons to walk amongst their animals from a young age on a regular basis, forming a positive relationship with their animals, will save them valuable time later on when handling them (Cooke, 2014; Francisco *et al.*, 2012). Getting cattle used to different areas, such as squeeze chutes, before they are needed to be handled fully or have an aversive procedure performed, are much easier to handle in this situation than if they are experiencing it for the first time. They also show lower stress levels, which is reflected in a reduced cortisol level (Andrade *et al.*, 2001). Stockpersons are the best people to speak to, to gain an understanding of the individual's temperament, and their advice should be taken while gaining the history of the animal.

9.2.5 Cattle Signals to Look For

When working with any cattle it is important that you have a good understanding of their behaviour and learn to read their body language. The emotional state of a cow can be expressed through its behaviour, so having a good knowledge of some of the signals to look for is key. The majority of signals will be displayed as a threat and it is only if this threat is ignored will physical contact be made. Bulls will show their aggression by pawing at the ground, lowering and rubbing the neck and shoulders on the ground. They will also stand side on to show their size. Remember, a bull can very quickly change from being very passive to highly aggressive, especially when there are cows around. Cows will also show aggression through pawing at the ground, lowering the head towards the ground and staring at the handler head on. They can also be heard to produce a snorting noise by expelling large amounts of air through their nose. Vocalization in cattle can be a sign of stress (Grandin, 2001). Cattle will also hold their heads up high if they are feeling threatened as they are on high alert. Holding the head high is way of looking for predators. Anxious and alert cattle are also likely to have large whites of the eyes and flared nostrils. The swishing of the tail or holding it upright into the air can both be a sign of agitation. Paying attention to the ears of the cow can tell you what it is reacting to and what draws its attention, as well as what mood it may be in. Cattle with a high anxiety level are likely to have diarrhoea, which can cause flooring to become slippery, so extra care must be taken.

9.3 How to Approach and Move Cattle

Successful handling relies on preparation. Clear instructions are required when moving cattle and each person involved needs to know the plan to ensure correct pressure is applied in the flight zone. When approaching either an individual or a group of cattle, the handler must make their presence known before entering the flight zone. This can be achieved by talking or giving a low call towards the cattle and moving slowly but purposefully, within the cows' field of vision. During all movement of cattle, the principle of pressure and release should be used; once an individual or group has moved away from the handler, the handler should remove themselves from the flight zone as a reward. Pressure is reapplied as needed. Handling with minimum disturbance reduces any unnecessary stress on cattle. Impatient handling causes injury and excessive force should always be avoided. It must be remembered that limited force is required to move the cattle and excessive force will increase the time for any animal to move along a chute or along a path (Goonewardene *et al.*, 1999).

9.3.1 Approaching and Moving a Group of Cattle

A group of cattle should be moved together as one group, using the collective flight zone and point of balance. When moving a group of cattle, if a leader can be identified within a group and a good working relationship between that individual cow and a stockperson is evident, this should be used where possible. This can significantly reduce the need to push cattle from behind. Where this is not possible, having two or more people working in a semicircular motion behind the cattle, is advised. Using the collective group flight zone, guide the cattle along a fence line or wall without using too much noise or aversive movements, such as hitting or slapping the cattle on the hindquarters. Allow the cattle to set their own pace and respect this. Be aware that continuous pushing from the rear of a group will rarely speed movement up, especially if more subordinate animals are being asked to get closer to the dominant individuals. If subordinate individuals are pressured too much, they will not look at where they walk but rather concentrate on where the dominant individuals are and how to escape them. This can cause them to hold their heads up high, meaning injuries between and within cattle will occur. Other signs to be aware off that might indicate that a group is pressured too much or incorrectly are cattle moving across the group from one side to the other, cattle pushing into each other and holding their heads either high or low towards the ground, and their eyes will be wide, so that the whites may be seen. If cattle are moved too quickly within a yard, they are likely to take corners too tightly. This can lead to bruising, as they might knock themselves on gate posts or walls, and it can increase the potential for lameness if they were to slip or fall over. Be careful with areas that are known to be slippery under foot and around corners to prevent this.

Trying to separate calves from their mothers or a smaller group from the remaining herd can be difficult due to the herding instincts. Care must be taken for both the handler and the animals involved. It is best to have at least two people involved in this situation, so that one person can guide the cattle towards a gate that the other person can open as the correct animal approaches. If a sorting gate is available this should be used.

The use of sticks to encourage cattle to move forward should be replaced with equipment such as flags, which are just as effective at moving cattle forward. Cattle see wider implements such as flags better than thin sticks, so are more likely to respond appropriately. This apparatus should only be used to guide the animal and not to hit or strike the animal or to cause fear. The Welfare of Farmed Animals (England) Regulations state '*No person shall apply an electric current to any animals for the purposes of immobilisation*'. Goads and electric prods should not be used. Goonewardene *et al.* (1999) found that cattle which received the electric prod on a regular basis reacted negatively to this. The maximum force required to move cattle along the chute increased and the time it took for any animal to move along the chute increased.

9.3.2 Approaching and Moving the Individual

Individual cattle should be moved using the same principles as a group, with pressure and release being applied as needed. Some cattle may have become used to human contact, so their flight zone may be incredibly small or even non-existent. Some of these cattle may have been trained to walk on halter and this may be the easier and preferred way of moving them. The cow should be encouraged to walk forward from the side and not dragged from the front end.

Cattle that are not halter trained but have a small flight zone may need a little more pressure applied to encourage them forward. This can be in the simple form of a gentle hand on the shoulder or rump, or a low hum and gentle encouragement by voice. Avoid using loud noises and shouting, as this may cause a group to move and not just the individual, or it may cause the animal to be startled and slip. In extreme cases where the cow may still not move forward, the tail can be lifted gently and pulled to the side until some resistance is felt (Figure 9.2). Overtwisting or incorrect twisting of the tail can lead

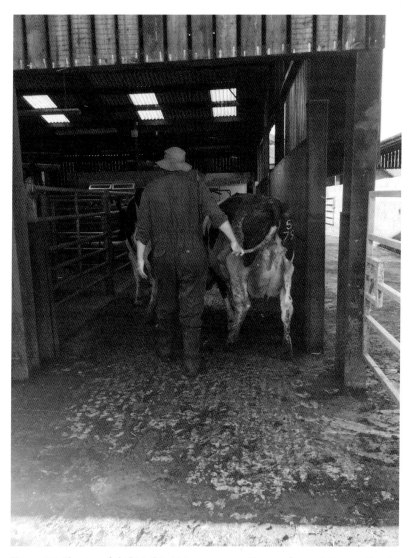

Figure 9.2 The use of slight tail twist to encourage the cow forward (Source: Courtesy of Reaseheath College).

to it breaking. Twisting of the tail and slapping the cow on the back end are highly aversive tactics and should be avoided as much as possible.

If a calf needs to be separated out from its mother, or a smaller group needs to be separated out from the remaining herd, this can be difficult due to their natural herding instincts. Care must be taken for both the handler and the animals involved. It is best to have at least two people involved in this situation and the entire group or both mother and calf are brought into a special separating area. This will allow one person to guide a few cattle at a time or just the mother cow towards a gate, and then a second person to open the gate as the correct animal(s) approach(es), shutting the gate before another animal can go through. If a sorting gate is available this should be used. Many dairy farms have an automated sorting gate to move cattle around into the correct lactation and feeding group. These are most efficient and stress free choices for such a task.

9.3.3 Moving a Calf

Calves will naturally follow their mother. If the mother and calf need to remain together, the focus can be placed on moving the cow as described previously for moving an individual. If the calf is to be separated from its mother, follow the procedure described previously and then guide the calf to the new area by placing one hand around the neck and chest area and the other hand behind the tail. This way the calf can be encouraged forward from the tail end and guided with the front end. Walk alongside the calf in a calm and confident manner. The calf is likely to be highly aroused as it is led away from the mother, so any path should be clear to allow for a smooth movement. Do not be tempted to grasp the tail or to pull the tail of the calf to control it, as this is highly aversive.

If a calf is small enough, it may be carried by one person by placing one hand around the neck and chest area and the other arm over the top of the calf and wrapped around the flank area. If the calf is too large for this, two people can link arms around the neck and abdomen of the calf and lift the calf. Calves that will not walk and are too heavy to carry, can be transported in either a wheel barrow or other form of transport (Figure 9.3). If this method is used, it is very important that the legs of the animal do not hang down over the sides, as this can cause broken limbs. It is best to tie the legs together with a slip knot and this will reduce the chances of the calf struggling and injuring itself.

Never carry or transport a calf upside down.

9.4 Handling Facilities

All facilities used for handling cattle should be safe to use and fit for purpose in order to reduce stress and ensure welfare. Facilities that are suitable for dairy cattle may not be suitable for beef cattle and vice versa. They should be designed from the perspective of the cow, with consideration given to how cattle move through the system. It is important that, within all handling facilities, any distractions are removed. These can include wire or string hanging down from the ceiling, clothing or material hanging on the sides, or changes in light, such as shadows or light coming through small gaps in the sides of pens. These can all cause cattle to balk and increase arousal level in all animals using the facilities. Reflections in any standing water or from metal flooring should also be removed as far as is possible. The use of padding for steel or wooden pens is suggested,

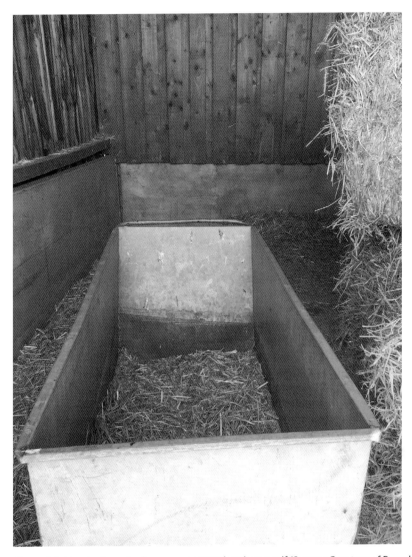

Figure 9.3 Livestock carrier for a young animal such as a calf (Source: Courtesy of Reaseheath College).

as this is less noisy for cattle and can reduce the number of reflections. Changes in type or quality of flooring can also stop an animal moving forward. Consideration to the slope of the floor should be considered, too. If these things are present and cannot be removed or changed at the time of handling, extra caution and patience with the animals is required to allow them time to process the information coming from their environment. This can help reduce the stress levels and keep the arousal level of the cattle low.

Cattle are good learners and if facilities are not set up correctly and cows escape, they will remember this and will keep escaping from that same point. All facilities should be kept clean and clear of any obstacles or projections that could harm or hinder the movement of cattle, or interfere with the handler. They should be placed in areas where

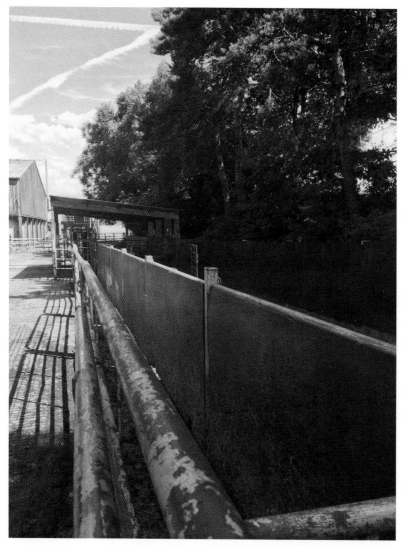

Figure 9.4 A handling facility for cattle. Note the shelter provided by the tress and the specially designed shelter at the end. Also note the holding facility has solid walls with one side made from wood to reduce the nose level of the metal barriers (Source: Courtesy of Reaseheath College).

cattle would not be exposed to extreme weather conditions or shelter should be provided (Figure 9.4). Remember, good facilities reduce time and labour for producers and avoid unnecessary stress and injury to the cattle.

When gathering cattle from the field or from the housing, they should be bought into a **crowding area**. This crowding area should have a place that protects the animals from extreme weather, as in Figure 9.4. It is important that this area allows cattle to move and turn around with sufficient space to prevent slipping and is not overcrowded. If it is only half-full with animals it will allow for subordinate individuals to avoid dominant animals, thereby reducing stress levels and potential injuries. Before moving cattle into the chute or race, they should be given 20–30 minutes to settle down in the crowding area, particularly if arousal levels are high. Crowd gates can be a useful method of encouraging cattle to move forwards into the next area; however, they should not be used to force the cattle but to just follow behind and should not make contact with the cow. Cattle must be allowed to move at their own pace to allow them to inspect the environment they are being asked to go into. Do not apply excessive pressure, as this will increase arousal and make handling more difficult.

A crowding area should be designed so that it slowly reduces in size as it guides cattle towards the entrance of the **chute** (this can be seen in Figure 9.4). Movement should be uphill and floors should be non-slip and maintained so that they are in good condition. This will encourage the group to move in single file. A circular area is best for encouraging continued forward movement but a funnel-shaped area into the chute is a good alternative. Curved, single-file chutes with solid walls work best for encouraging cattle to continue to walk forward as they follow the leader of the group. It is important that this curve is not too long and that they can see daylight in front of them or space to walk into, or else they may try to turn back if they can only see a solid wall in front of them. Curved chutes tend to fill up faster, quicker and more efficiently than straight races. Providing a chute that is V-shaped will also help to guide cattle forward and help to prevent slipping or falling in an area. A gate that prevents too many cattle moving into the chute at once will also help to prevent cattle from slipping or balking too much. Avoid moving cattle into direct sunlight, as they cannot see the area they are moving into. Also avoid moving cattle from a very light area to a very dark area and vice versa as this can cause them to balk. They cannot judge the level of flooring at this change in light. If using a straight chute, make sure handlers are not visible ahead of the cow, as they will be at the incorrect point of balance and the cow will not continue to walk forward. The end of the chute should lead to the **squeeze chute** and **head gate** (Figures 9.5 and 9.6) for restraint.

Special sorting gates should be set up so that when sorting cattle, this can be carried out with little interference. Sort calves from cows and bulls from cows and remove excitable animals, so that they are disturbed the least when handling others. Quiet animals should be separated away from nervous animals rather than vice versa.

New **roundhouse buildings** incorporate the handling facilities within the house itself. The handling pen is in the middle of the house and allows the cattle to enter from their own resting area and be sorted before being returned to a resting area. There is less need for moving cattle large distances and the housing environment does not change too much.

9.4.1 Special Note: Bulls and Calves; Use of Dogs and Vehicles

Special consideration needs to be given when handling bulls. Bulls, whether they are dairy or beef, can be highly dangerous and can cause severe damage and, potentially, death. Bulls are territorial and defensive of their space, which should always be respected when moving an individual. Bulls reared in isolation are likely to be more dangerous than animals reared as a group. Take note of the threat signals previously described in this chapter and respect the size and power of the bull. **NEVER** turn your back on a bull or make any sudden movement. If you have a good understanding of animal behaviour, you as a handler can predict the action of an animal and direct an appropriate response that leads to effective and humane handling before the situation escalates.

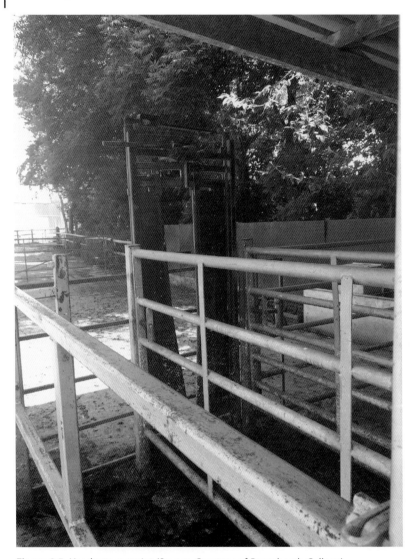

Figure 9.5 Headgate restraint (Source: Courtesy of Reaseheath College).

Female cattle can be highly protective of their young and can be as dangerous as a bull when with their calves. The cows' behaviour should be noted when handling them in this situation and, as with bulls, the signals of any stress or aggression must be respected. When handling cows with calves at foot, dogs should be removed from the area, as cows will become more protective of their young when dogs are around. Young calves can normally be haltered or handled easily when away from the mother by guiding them from the head and back end.

Vehicles can be used to help move dangerous cattle, such as bulls or young, inexperienced cattle that may be highly aroused. Well trained dogs that are calm and quiet around cattle can also be used to aid the handler when moving groups of

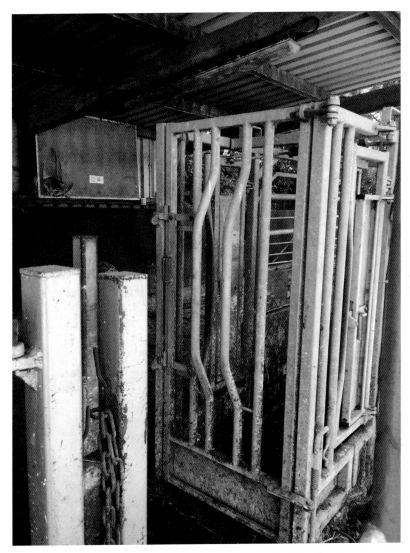

Figure 9.6 Headgate restraint (Source: Courtesy of Reaseheath College).

cattle if a handler is on their own. The cattle should be used to dogs, which should only be used to guide cattle in from an open space into an enclosed area. Once the cattle are enclosed, the dog should be restrained, so as not to avoid provoking too much arousal. Poorly trained dogs can cause a group to scatter, creating a very stressful environment for all involved. Care must be taken when using either a vehicle or a dog, so that excessive pressure is not placed onto the cattle and that they are allowed to move at their own pace. Be as patient as you would be on foot. Excessive pressure with the use of either a dog or vehicle will likely increase the arousal level and, thus, danger of aggression. Rushing cattle will increase the chances of lameness occurring and other injuries.

9.5 How to Restrain Cattle

The degree of restraint required for each animal will depend on the individuals' temperament, age and previous handling experience. Use the minimal amount of restraint required by each animal to reduce stress.

9.5.1 Physical Restraint

When full physical restraint is required, cattle should be herded into the chute from the crowding pen and walked up into the **squeeze chute**. Squeeze chutes consist of a headgate, a tailgate or back bar and removable side panels (Figures 9.7 and 9.8). The gate can be operated either manually or controlled with hydraulics. The squeeze chute is designed to hold each animal individually ready for restraint. A squeeze chute that has V-shaped sides will help to support the cattle, keeping them calmer, so reducing the chances of the individual falling. Removable side panels should be located immediately behind the headgate to allow veterinarians and handlers access to the side of the cow to administer care at the side of the animal.

The **headgate** is designed to hold the head of the cow once it reaches this section. Headgates can be self-catching, which close automatically (Figure 9.9). These are often found in pens in which animals rest and feed. This can make the experience of being restrained less stressful, as they do not need to be moved out of their home environments. This type of headgate should only be used for minor procedures that do not require the full body of the cow to be restrained.

Headgates can also be a scissors–stanchion design, which consists of two halves that pivot at the bottom (Figure 9.5), or full-opening stanchion, which has two halves that work like a pair of sliding doors (Figures 9.6, 9.7 and 9.10). Small operators are more likely to have self-catching or full-opening headgates. Adding a nose bar prevents cattle moving their heads up and down whilst in the chute. When cattle exit a chute, they do so quickly, so ensure non-slip clear areas for them to move to.

Some cattle can be restrained by simply being placed into an area where they are unable to turn around or move forward and backwards, such as in an artificial insemination (AI) pen (Figure 9.11). Note that in this area the cattle are prevented from moving backwards with the use of a simple chain across the back of the pen, and they are unable to move forward due to the wall. Holding cattle in an area such as this can allow for minor procedures, such as AI, to be carried out without having to restrain the cattle with excessive pressure. Providing an area such as this where a number of individuals can be held together can reduce stress. This also provides a good space for training younger more naïve animals to get used to an area by pairing them with a more experienced, calm adult cow.

If a cow is prone to kicking in this area, either the tail can be gently lifted or a rope can be placed around the abdomen area with the free end passing through a loop and then tied to a side bar of the holding pen or squeeze chute. When the cow goes to kick, as she arches her back, pressure will be applied through the rope reducing the chances of her kicking. Caution must be taken to not apply the rope too tightly, it should simply fit snuggly around the abdomen.

Some cattle and calves may be halter trained and for minor procedures or movement of cattle this may be all that is needed. The most common type of halter is a **rope** halter;

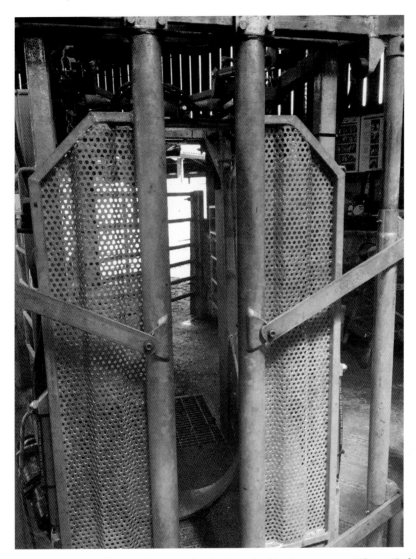

Figure 9.7 Squeeze chute. This example also has a backing bar to prevent the cattle from moving backwards and is designed to be used when trimming cattle's feet (Source: Courtesy of Reaseheath College).

however, they can be made out of a variety of materials (Figures 9.12 and 9.13). A **rope halter** can also be used for extra control of the head during restraint in a headgate.

Halters should be made ready with an enlarged head piece and nose loop. To place a halter on to the cow follow these steps:

1) Make sure that the halter is opened up so that enough space is provided in the nose and head loops to place them easily onto the cow.
2) Drop the enlarged head piece over the poll (Figure 9.14) and move the enlarged nose piece down towards the nose.

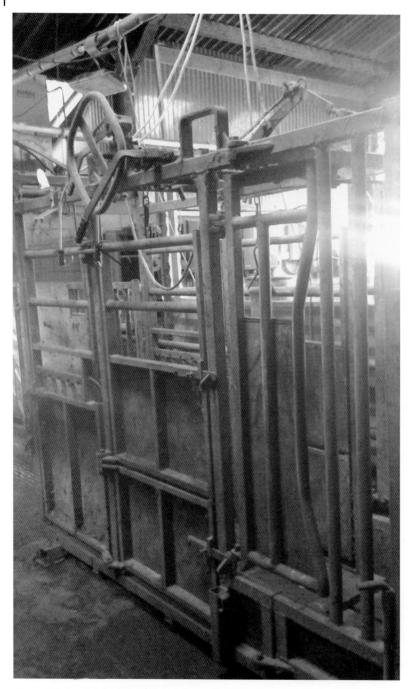

Figure 9.8 Another example of a squeeze chute showing the removal sides for access to the cow (Source: Courtesy of Krista McLennan, 2016).

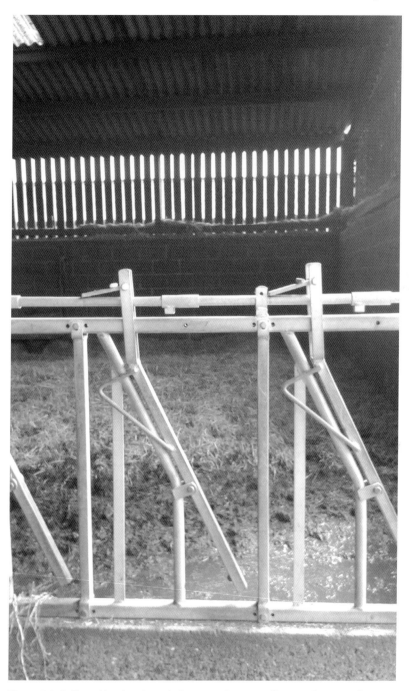

Figure 9.9 Self-catching headgate in home environment (Source: Courtesy of Krista McLennan, 2016).

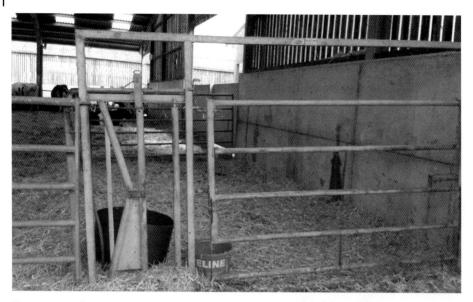

Figure 9.10 Full opening stanchion (Source: Courtesy of Krista McLennan, 2016).

3) Place the nose piece over the nose and pull it towards you so that the halter fits snuggly (Figure 9.15). Do not pull the rope too tightly, as this may be aversive to the cow and could startle her.

The key points to remember when using a halter are confinement, patience, keep moving with the animal and leave the halter on a slack lead rope until the last moment. The proper placement of a halter is key to ensuring full control. Traditionally, cattle are led from the left, so the halter should be placed so that the lead exits from the left, from the chin area. This will allow the head to turn and for the handler to have full control. If the halter were upside down, the lead would exit from behind the ear and the animal could turn the nose away from the restraint.

Where extra control is required, such as when handling a bull that is over 12 months of age, a nose ring can be applied. Rings should be fitted well forward of the nasal septum cartilage. Attachments to the nose rings such an extra lead rope are also possible to provide further restraint (Figure 9.16). Rope that is attached to a nose ring should never be tied.

In other cattle where extra control may be required, pressure can be applied to the nasal septum by holding the septum distal to the cartilage for a few seconds between thumb and forefinger. If this needs to be carried out for a longer period of time, the use of a nose holder is recommended. The nose holder should have rounded smooth bulbous ends, with a 3 mm gap between ends and a device for keeping them closed without being held. **Do not** leave the animal unattended when these are being used. Damage to the sensitive tissue can occur if the holder's finger pressure is used incorrectly or in an overzealous fashion.

Smaller cattle such as calves can be restrained by placing them onto their sides. To do this the calf should be stood parallel to the handler. Reach over the top of the calf and grasp the back leg that is nearest to the handler and with the other hand reach between

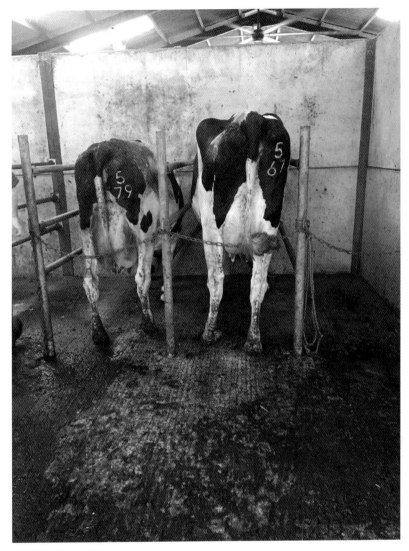

Figure 9.11 AI pen (Source: Courtesy of Reaseheath College).

the front legs to grasp the front leg that is nearest to the handler. Gently lifting both these legs so that the calf is placed off balance, allow the calf to gently slide down the leg of the handler. Once the calf is in this position an assistant can hold the calf by placing a knee onto the shoulder area and holding down the front and back legs that are now most prominent. If an assistant is not able to help, the front and back legs can be tied together.

Other forms of restraint are available depending upon the type of procedure that is being carried out. Tilting tables can offer complete restraint and are often used when foot trimming cattle. The tables can be mobile or fixed, they can restrain the head and girth area and can use winches and ropes to prevent cattle from kicking (see Section 9.5.2). It is unknown how stressful these types of restraint can be, so cattle should not be held for

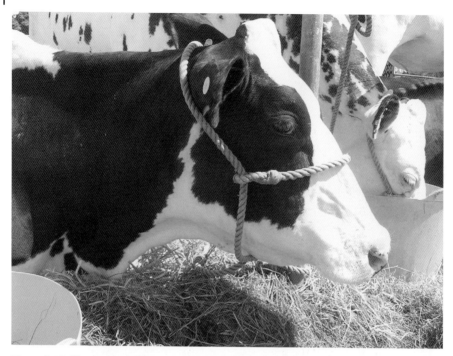

Figure 9.12 Classic rope halter on an adult cow (Source: Courtesy of Krista McLennan, 2016).

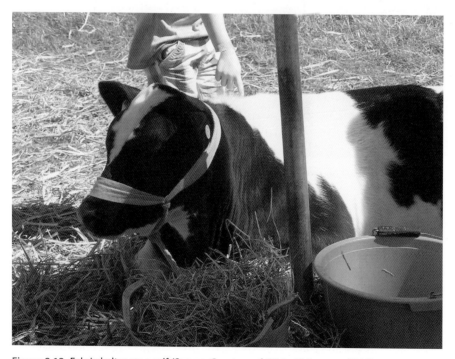

Figure 9.13 Fabric halter on a calf (Source: Courtesy of Krista McLennan, 2016).

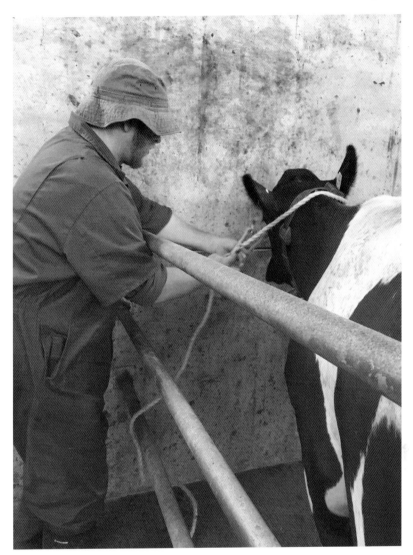

Figure 9.14 Place the head collar over the top of the poll and move the nose piece down towards the nose (Source: Courtesy of Reaseheath College).

any longer than 30 minutes in this position. This will also prevent the build-up of gas in the gut.

9.5.2 Roping or Casting

Most farms will now have specialized handling facilities; however, on smaller farms or small holdings special facilities may not be available. Makeshift restraint areas may be possible, where a gate is fitted to a solid wall and the gate can be moved so that the cattle can be held between the gate and the wall. Where this is not possible, the animal may need to be casted or roped to help restrain it or to reduce the chances of being kicked.

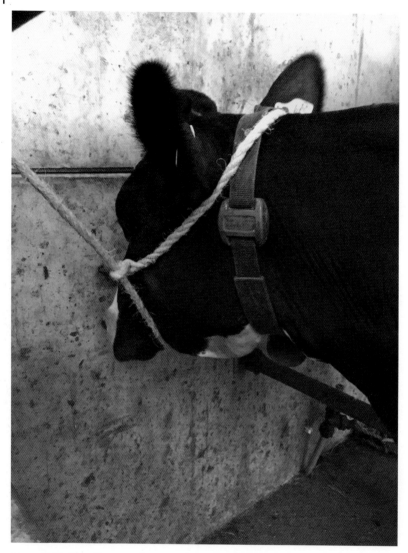

Figure 9.15 Place the nose piece over the nose and pull the end of the rope towards you such that it fits snuggly to the cow (Source: Courtesy of Reaseheath College).

To restrain the cow with ropes the following can be employed:

- **Leg tie** – The tying of legs can be used to both reduce the chance of being kicked as well as a method of restraint. The simplest form of leg restraint is through the use of shackles or using a rope, making a figure of eight between the two back legs down around the pastern area. To hold up a front leg, place a loop of rope around the pastern of the leg that you wish to raise. Pass the rope over the top of the withers. Whilst pulling on this rope, push the cow slightly at the shoulder to move her balance on to the alternative front leg. This will allow you to lift the front leg more easily. A back leg can be lifted manually by reaching from the inside of the thigh and sliding the hand

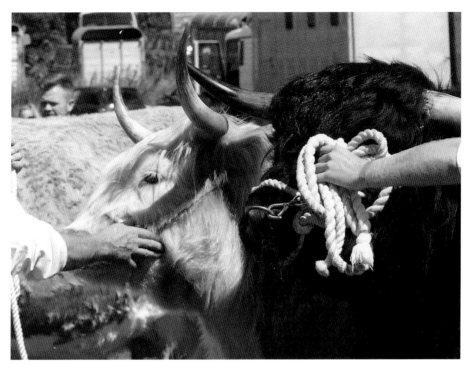

Figure 9.16 A nose ring on a bull that has a lead attached for extra control along with a traditional rope head collar (Source: Courtesy of Krista McLennan, 2016).

down the front of the leg pushing on it once the pastern is reached. This, however, can be dangerous, as cattle can quickly move their back legs in an upwards and forwards arc. This method should only be used if the cow is used to this and is restrained at the head with a head collar and lead rope.

- If the cow needs to be restrained further through the use of ropes, a **Burley Hitch** can be used. Place a long length of rope with its centre over the withers. Pass the free ends through the front legs of the cow and cross them over at this point. Pass them back over the back of the cow and then through the back legs. Care must be taken at this point to not catch up the udder or penis and testicles; they should be placed out of the way and the ropes should touch the inside of the legs. When the ends of the rope are pulled, the cow should go down into lateral recumbency. The direction of the fall can be controlled by pulling on the rope in the direction required. The free ends can now be used to tie the rear leg in place by keeping the rope taught and passing it around a flexed leg at the pastern joint. The rope is then passed back around the leg in a figure of eight to keep the rope taught. As this method causes the cattle to fall, care must be taken to ensure the safety of all handlers and animals involved. This should only be performed in an area that has a soft surface, such as a straw yard or field. It should **NEVER** be performed in a concreted area.
- The **rope squeeze** is the standard method of casting a cow. Place a loop of rope over the neck of the cattle. Pass the free end over the back of the cow and reach under the sternum to retrieve it. Leaving a length of rope that runs along the back just past the

shoulder, pass the free end through this loop, forming a half-hitch. Repeat this process again so that the second half hitch is just in front of the udder. Once the rope is pulled, the cow will lie down in sternal recumbency. The back legs can be restrained as described in the previous section. Care must be taken when using this method that the milk vein of female cows and the penis of male cows is not damaged by the rope under the abdomen. Any procedure requiring this cast should be performed as quickly as possible so that the cattle can be released.

- Cattle may also benefit from the addition of a mask during handling to cover their eyes. This can reduce the stress levels experienced. Cattle that were **blindfolded** whilst in a squeeze chute had a decrease in respiratory rate, decrease in heart rate and a reduced cortisol levels when compared to cattle that did not have a blindfold on (Andrade *et al.*, 2001).

9.6 Training for Restraint

Exposure to novel environments on a regular basis can help prepare cattle. It is good practice to have animals acclimatized to any new sights and sounds in a safe environment before they are exposed to it for restraint. The naturally inquisitive nature of cattle should be used and consideration should be given to allow them to approach new things at their own pace rather than forcing them. Forcing the cow is more likely to install a negative memory rather than a positive one, which can be formed when cattle are allowed to explore for themselves.

Cattle can be trained to come to call. This is using the natural behaviour of following the leader of the group. A good stockperson can train the cattle so that they see them as the leader. The best time to do this is when feeding cattle. Produce the same call or signal to the cattle when giving them feed. They will respond better to this if it is completed at the same time each day and preferably in the cooler parts of the day, taking advantage of their diurnal nature.

9.7 Special Considerations

- The majority of accidents occur when unsympathetic handling has taken place and planning has been poor. Poor handling results in negative experiences for both the cattle and the handler, and welfare and productivity are reduced.
- A swishing tail can cause significant damage to a handler. During handling procedures where the tail may be a nuisance, it can be tied out of the way onto the body. It should never be tied to a static fixture.
- Downer cattle should be considered with great care. Cattle must be given time to stand on their own. If support is needed, it should be provided in the most safe and effective manner.
- Cattle have extremely good memories and will associate a handler with the treatment they give out.
- Cattle can kick in a forward, outwards and backwards arc. This means that they can reach someone standing at their shoulder. Always stand in a safe place when working with cattle.

Key Points

- Always make sure that cattle are aware of your approach before you reach the flight zone to avoid surprising the cow and causing it to balk. This can be performed by making gentle humming noises or walking into the line of vision before entering their flight zone.
- Make use of the cattle's natural flight zone to move an individual as well as a group, using the principle of pressure and release.
- All movements around cattle should be slow and deliberate, and handlers should remain calm and patient. Avoid loud noises such as yelling and any aversive techniques such as tail twisting or rump slapping. Rushing cattle causes slips, falls and bruising, which are all indicators of poor welfare.
- Keep animals together as a group or at least in a pair to avoid isolation. Separate calves out from mothers, and bulls away from females.
- Preparations for movement should be made in advance, removing all distractions from the environment and any sharp objects.
- Make use of experienced personal and stockpersons who handle the cattle on a daily basis – they will know the cattle well.
- Most accidents are down to not understanding or respecting the behaviour signals that are displayed by the cattle.
- Remember, give cattle time to move at their own pace. Slower is often quicker in the case of moving livestock.

Self-assessment Questions

1 What is the flight zone?

2 Describe what optimal pressure means.

3 Describe how to restrain a calf.

4 Why use curved chutes?

5 Where is the point of balance?

Answers can be found in the back of the book.

References

Andrade, O., Orihuela, A., Solano, J. and Galina, C.S. (2001) Some effects of repeated handling and the use of a mask on stress responses in zebu cattle during restraint. *Applied Animal Behaviour Science*, **71** (3), 175–181.

Cooke, R.F. (2014) Bill E. Kunkle Interdisciplinary Beef Symposium: Temperament and acclimation to human handling influence growth, health and reproductive responses in *Bos Taurus* and *Bos indicus* cattle. *Journal of Animal Science*, **92** (12), 5325–5333.

Francisco, C.L., Cooke, R.F., Marques, R.S. *et al.* (2012) Effects of temperament and acclimation to handling on feedlot performance of *Bos Taurus* feeder cattle originated from a rangeland-based cow-calf system. *Journal of Animal Science*, **90** (13), 5067–5077.

Goonewardene, L.A., Price, M.A., Okine, E. and Berg, R.T. (1999) Behavioural responses to handling and restraint in dehorned and polled cattle. *Applied Animal Behaviour Science*, **64** (3), 159–167.

Grandin, T. (2001) Cattle vocalisations are associated with handling and equipment problems at beef slaughter plants. *Applied Animal Behaviour Science*, **71** (3), 191–201.

McTavish, E.J., Decker, J.E., Schnabel, R.D. *et al.* (2013) New World cattle show ancestry from multiple independent domestication events. *Proceedings of the National Academy of Sciences of the USA*, **110** (15), E1398.

Further Reading

Grandin, T. (ed) (2015) *Improving Animal Welfare. A Practical Approach*, 2nd edn, CABI (Centre for Agriculture and Biosciences International), Wallingford, UK.

10

Handling and Restraint of Small Ruminants

Krista M. McLennan[1] and Stella J. Chapman[2]

[1]Chester University, Chester, UK
[2]University Centre Hartpury, Gloucestershire, UK

Sheep (*Ovis aries*) were one of the first mammals to be domesticated by humans; however, the exact timeline of events has been unclear. The use of mitochondrial DNA testing has recently made it possible to trace back the ancestry of many animals, including cattle, horses, pigs and goats, and evidence suggests that the number of wild progenitors for these species is limited. With sheep this is not the case and it is thought that a large number of wild ancestral species and subspecies exist (Hiendleder *et al.*, 2002). Archaeological findings have traced the sheep back to 11 000 and 9000 BC in Mesopotamia, with the most common hypothesis being that *Ovis aries* descended from the Asiatic (*Ovis orientalis*) species of mouflon. Many studies have looked at the ancestry of sheep and there has been conflicting evidence with regards to the numbers of ancestors. It is now thought that three major groups of Eurasian wild sheep (mouflon, urial and argali) are the ancestors of the domestic sheep and it is these groups that are believed to have contributed to specific breeds (Hiendleder *et al.*, 2002).

Sheep were originally kept for their meat, milk and hides. Selection for 'woolly' sheep is thought to have begun around 6000 BC, with wool being spun by 5000 BC. The main centre for wool production in antiquity was Central Asia and the 'wool industry' was one of the first ways in which trade was established between different countries.

Like sheep, the goat (*Capra hircus*) was domesticated by man early in history from its wild ancestor *Capra aegargus*. The origins of the goat, as with many other species, is, however, uncertain and controversial. Archaeological evidence suggests that Neolithic farmers in the Near East started keeping small herds of goats around 10 000–11 000 years ago for their meat, milk and hides (Luikart *et al.*, 2001). The fact that there is enormous morphological diversity amongst the more than 300 goat breeds found today would support multiple domestication events and goats are the most adaptable and geographically widespread livestock species. Luikart *et al.* (2001) found using phylogeographic analysis that goat populations are less genetically structured than cattle populations; this weak structuring suggests extensive intercontinental transport of goats and that goats may have played an important role in human migration and commerce. Goats continue to remain the main economic resource in many developing countries and, in the west, have become of growing economic importance for their meat and milk.

10.1 Behaviour

Sheep and goats are both highly sociable animals. They are prey species, so live as a group to protect themselves against predators. This flocking instinct is very strong in sheep. A sheep that becomes separated from the remaining group will become increasingly anxious and will be highly motivated to regain contact with the group. This can lead to sheep becoming dangerous to both themselves and to handlers, as they may attempt to jump fences or other barriers, which can lead to breaking of legs or escape from the fields onto road or other unintended areas. Whilst goats have this instinct to group, it is not as strong as it is for sheep; goats will try to remain with the group but have a higher tendency to split off from a group than sheep.

As prey species, sheep and goats, like cattle, have a good sense of vision and hearing. Their eyes are on the side of their head, allowing them to monitor their surrounding environments, with a small blind spot towards the rear. Having eyes on the side of their head means that they do not have good depth perception, except for directly in front of them. This can cause them to startle when objects suddenly appear at their sides. This also explains why sheep and goats may balk at changes in their pathway and subsequently lower their heads, so that they are able to use their binocular vision to assess the distraction. Understanding the visual perception of sheep and goats is important to the design of handling facilities.

The behaviour of sheep and goats will differ due to the different rearing and management systems employed. Goats are often kept for milk in the United Kingdom and are often used to being handled. They are highly inquisitive animals and are likely to approach a handler that they may have formed a bond with, such as an owner. Their friendly behaviour can make them easier to handle. However, if handled incorrectly, they will soon learn how to avoid being caught. Sheep, on the other hand, are handled less, as they are primarily reared for meat and kept out at grass on lowland farms or out on the hills on hill farms. Sheep will try to keep a safe distance from humans and can be flighty by nature. This, and the lack of handling, can make catching and restraining them more difficult. Sheep have very good long term memories, especially for aversive handling, and can remember certain people. If they are handled incorrectly they will also do their best to avoid being caught and can even cause an entire group to scatter when rounding up.

It must be remembered that each animal is an individual, so will respond differently to the catching and restraint procedures. Different breeds of the sheep or goat have different temperaments and an animals' previous experience can change their response. Observing sheep or goats before handling can alert you to any potential danger, as well as allow you to assess the temperament of the animal before making a final judgement on how best to handle that individual. Some important signs to watch for include: the ears of a sheep, they can indicate the state of mind of the animal and can indicate the direction of any distractions; pawing at the ground or stamping at the ground, which can indicate that the animal is not comfortable with the proximity of the handler; the head down or throwing the head around can suggest fear or aggression; and grinding of teeth may be heard if an animal becomes distressed or agitated. High anxiety levels can increase the level of diarrhoea.

10.1.1   How to Use Behavioural Traits to Effect when Handling

10.1.1.1   The Flocking Instinct

The flocking instinct of sheep is an important trait that should be respected and used for effective and efficient handling. Sheep want to maintain visual contact with another sheep at all times. This applies at times of gathering and when handling. Keeping a flock together will keep all sheep much calmer and reduce the need for continued attempts to capture or restrain them. Even if only one sheep needs to be caught, gathering together a small group that contains that individual will make the process much smoother than if just one individual is moved on its own.

The principle of the flight zone and point of balance described for cattle applies to individual sheep and to the flock. The instinct to remain as a group in sheep means that the flock can be moved using this principle of pressure and release. It must be remembered that hill sheep will have a larger flight zone compared to sheep that are handled more often, so care must be taken not to pressure the sheep too much to ensure that they remain calm. Sheep show their unease by stamping their front legs or head butting. They may also show their fear by keeping their heads low to the ground and trying to move away from anyone trying to get hold of their chin. A calm flock of sheep is much easier and faster to move than a flock that is being pushed in an impatient manner. It can take 20–30 minutes for sheep to calm down. Remember, slower is faster.

An individual goat will maintain its own flight zone but this is likely to be very small when it has been handled well before. If a flight zone is penetrated too deeply for an individual it can become unpredictable and dangerous to handle. Signs that a goat is becoming uncomfortable are snorting, stamping and the hair along the spine and the tail raised. If warning signs are not heeded, the goat will try to head butt you or rear up.

10.1.1.2   Follow the Leader

Goats do not have the same herding instinct as sheep, so are likely to scatter if the same principles are applied to gather a group. However, the following instinct of goats is strong and can be used to effectively and efficiently handle goats. If a lead doe can be identified, catching and leading this doe into a holding pen will likely encourage the rest of the group to join her. This ability to use a lead doe can be very effective at keeping the animals calm and handling them effectively without needing force. Goats can also be easily trained to come to call, meaning that no pressure is needed to catch up the goats. Friendly, gentle handling of goats is a must to maintain this relationship; the earlier a relationship can be built between a goat and a stockperson, the easier it is to handle at a later stage (Boivin and Braastad, 1996; Boivin *et al.*, 2000). Good human–animal relationships built from early stage can be effective at fostering a positive handling environment and animal welfare. Even sheep can benefit from early positive human contact, as it can reduce timidity in lambs towards humans (Markowitz *et al.*, 1998). Hand-reared lambs or pet sheep will also often follow a handler, so the same principle of training a lead sheep can be applied as with goats, reducing the need to use pressure as a means of moving sheep. The use of an older, more experienced sheep or doe can be used to lead younger, less experienced sheep through a handling facility and to provide social support during restraint. Good gentle handling and the building of a relationship is vitally important to maintaining good handling procedures. It also has the potential to reduce subsequent pain sensitivity (Guesgen *et al.*, 2013), which could be key when handling and restraining an animal for common husbandry procedures that are painful.

10.2   How to Approach and Move Sheep

10.2.1   Methods and Equipment

Whenever moving or handling sheep, preparation is important. The instructions to all parties involved must be clear and the plans double-checked. Gates that need to be opened must be done so in advance, to avoid the sheep being pressured into a corner from which they cannot escape, and all possible unintended escape routes must be blocked off. The principles of pressure and release using the natural flight zone of the group, as well as of the individual, should be applied to sheep as they are in cattle. Sheep will follow one another and only gentle pressure is required from behind. They do not need to be rushed or forced to move forward. Loud noises, such as shouting or banging, and fast unpredictable movements are not required. The use of flags to encourage the animals forward or to redirect their movements is a useful way of increasing the pressure without increasing the stress levels and compromising the welfare of the sheep. Once a group is on the move and directed properly, it should move fluidly as one group. Too much pressure will cause smothering, whereby the sheep jump onto each other's back, compromising their welfare and potentially leading to injury.

10.2.2   Approaching and Moving a Group of Sheep

During a gather it is important to keep sheep together as one flock and use their natural flocking instinct (Figure 10.1).

As with the cattle, there is a collective flight zone and point of balance to the group. Handlers or dogs (see special considerations for using dogs to move sheep) should be worked in a semicircle behind the sheep, guiding them along a fence line or down a naturally drawn path. The group, under proper control, will move fluidly and easily into where is intended. Move them slowly and quietly so not to excite them. If any sheep break away from the main flock it is important to wait for them to join back with the main group. If you do not wait for the sheep to rejoin, more sheep will start to break away from the group to join the second group and the entire flock can end up being scattered again. Continued attempts at gathering the sheep can be exhausting to both the sheep and the handlers. If there are a few sheep lagging behind the rest of the flock, this could mean something is wrong with these sheep. The flock must be moved at the pace of those at the back to keep the group calm and together.

Special care must be taken when gathering in hill sheep to ensure that their welfare is not compromised. Gathering in flocks off the hills is only carried out a few times each year and the sheep are not used to human contact, making them more flighty. Ewes may have lambs at foot, so it is important that they are allowed to move at the pace of their lambs. If a ewe was to become separated from her lamb she will leave the main group to

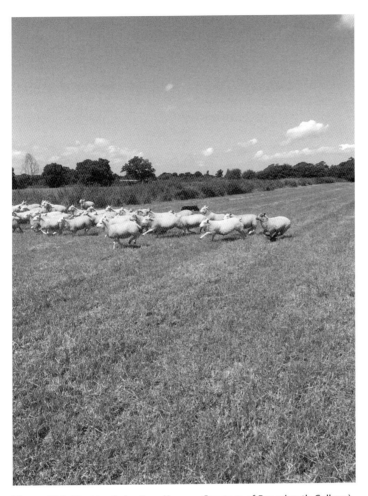

Figure 10.1 Flocking behaviour (Source: Courtesy of Reaseheath College).

gather the lamb, which can compromise the entire gather, scattering sheep across the hill. Gathering from across the hill can take a few hours and sheep must be allowed time to rest and move at their own pace. Consideration to weather conditions and terrain must be made, as both can make it more dangerous to rush sheep. The use of vehicles is now possible in this terrain but this can increase the speed at which the sheep may move. Take advantage of their natural want to remain with the group and allow them to follow at their own pace. Be aware that any sheep that have been recently gathered will be tired as well as having an increased arousal level. If handling after a gather, precaution needs to be taken. It is better to give the sheep time to rest for 30 minutes at least before performing any procedure.

When a group is being driven through a gateway, pressure must be eased, allowing the group to go through the entrance at its own pace. The entrance or gateway must also be big enough to avoid smothering or injury caused by being pushed against railings and so on. It is beneficial to have someone nearby such areas, so that they can step in and put pressure on to turn the group away if there is any risk of smothering.

If a small number of sheep are needed, they can be 'drafted' or 'cut' from the rest of the group with a very well trained dog. However, sometimes it is easier and less stressful to move the whole group into a handling yard from where they can be moved and separated out more easily with a separating gate at the end of a race.

Sheep have been known to be able to be trained to become leaders (Bremner *et al.*, 1980) and can be used to move a flock into a smaller space without needing to use pressure from behind. This improves the animal's welfare and is likely quicker than with dogs or human handlers.

10.2.3 Approaching and Moving an Individual Sheep

Sheep should be approached from behind when they are in a small enough space to ease capture; the chin should then be reached for. Sheep are effectively restrained by the head, by cupping your hand under the chin and gently lifting whilst using the other hand to support the back end (Figure 10.2).

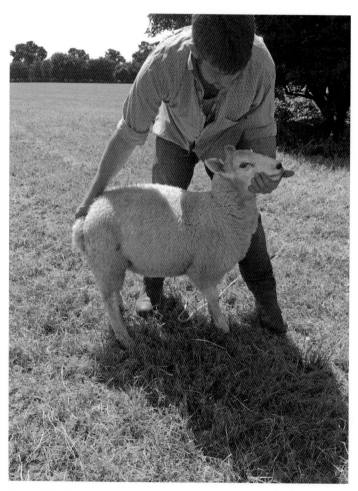

Figure 10.2 Simple restraint of standing sheep (Source: Courtesy of Reaseheath College).

Elevating the head slightly with a good grip under the chin and one hand behind is enough to move an individual sheep. Never grab a sheep by its tail or by the wool. Pulling on the wool is painful to the sheep, compromising its welfare. It can also cause bruising of the skin, which will result in the down-grading of a carcass.

The use of a crook around a back leg (Figure 10.3) is possible, too, but caution must be exercised when using this method and only experienced handlers should attempt this type of restraint. Severe injuries can occur if it is not performed correctly. The use of a crook around the neck is advised against, as it can cause severe damage.

Sheep with horns can be dangerous and holding the chin is not a safe way to handle these sheep long term. Once the sheep has been caught, one hand and then the other should be transferred to the horn. The horns should be held as close to the head as possible and not at the end, as this is likely to cause more damage due to excess force produced. Young sheep should not be handled by their horns, as long term damage can be caused if it is not performed correctly.

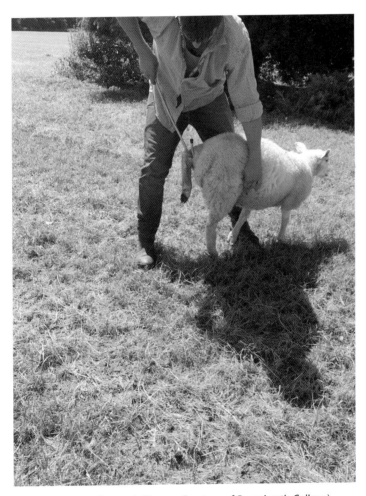

Figure 10.3 Use of a crook (Source: Courtesy of Reaseheath College).

10.2.4 Handling Facilities

Good handling facilities that have been designed from the sheep's perspective will make working with them much easier and less stressful for all involved. Consideration will have been made regarding the amount of space needed for the flock, the lighting of areas, the surface on which the sheep walk and the direction of travel, as well as to how easy they will be maintained and kept clean. Sheep should move steadily and with ease through the facilities with very little pressure being applied from the human. Dogs should not be used within the handling facilities themselves and should be secured outside of this area. Make sure that you are up to date with the relevant legal and recommended codes of practice.

All routes leading into and within the handling pens should be clear of any obstacles and all possible escape routes blocked. To reduce injury, routes and entrances into pens should be wide enough to allow a group through without squashing. The sides of any chutes or holding pens should be solid, so that animals feel safer and are not distracted by

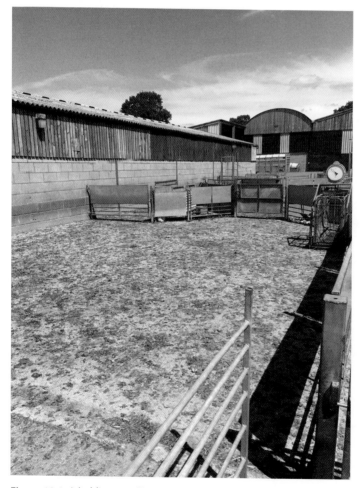

Figure 10.4 A holding pen (Source: Courtesy of Reaseheath College).

handlers or other objects outside the pen, bearing in mind that a sheep must maintain visual contact with another sheep at all times. There should be no sudden change of direction and corners should be smooth. Sharp turns and dead ends should be avoided, as they will prevent sheep from moving forward; a curved chute that allows the sheep to see others in front can work well in encouraging them to move forward. Sheep prefer to move from a darkened area towards a lighter area; however, contrasts in light should be avoided as much as possible.

The **holding pen** is an area where sheep can be held once they have been gathered in from the field or hill (Figure 10.4). This can either be a portable or solid construction within a yard. The pen should provide enough space to allow some movement of the flock without them climbing on each other's back, but small enough to restrict the sheep from moving too far away from the handler. When trying to catch a sheep in a larger area, the use of gates to reduce the available space is suggested. Portable gates or hurdles should be moved in a calm and effective manner to avoid startling the sheep.

From the holding pen, sheep should be guided into the race through the use of **forcing pen**. This may consist of a funnel-shaped pen that leads from the holding pen into the race itself or it may be curved and use a **swing** or **backing** gate to help guide a small number of sheep into the race. The forcing pen should be designed to ensure an even flow of sheep into the race, but it can also double as an area to catch a smaller flock of sheep once the main group is within the holding pen (Figures 10.5 and 10.6).

From the forcing pen the sheep can be encouraged into the **race or chute** in single file (Figures 10.7 and 10.8). Systems that allow sheep to maintain visual contact with the sheep in front, or for the lead sheep to see an open space, will keep the sheep moving forward through the race with ease. To avoid a sheep balking or turning within the race,

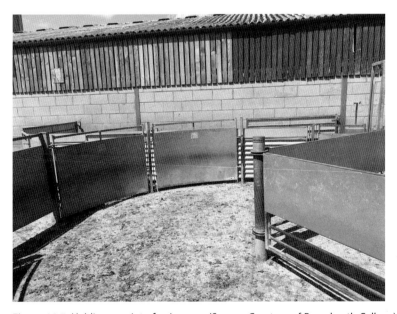

Figure 10.5 Holding pen into forcing pen (Source: Courtesy of Reaseheath College).

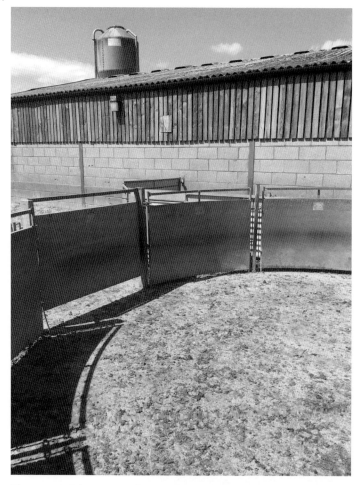

Figure 10.6 A forcing pen (Source: Courtesy of Reaseheath College).

it is important to keep all sheep within the race moving in the same direction as any sheep outside the race and for any other distractions to be removed. This may include objects over the sides, patches of light and shade occurring in breaks in the walls or even seeing a handler at the other end of the chute or race. Solid sides to a chute help to obscure some of these distractions and also prevent legs from getting stuck. The sides of the race should be high enough to prevent the sheep from jumping out and the race should be narrow enough to prevent the sheep from turning around. The use of backing gates can be useful to slow the passage of individuals through the race, preventing a build-up of sheep as well as preventing an animal escaping by going backwards. If they are to be used, there should only be one near to the end of the race and should allow three or four sheep in the space at a time. A sorting gate may be located at the end of the race; this will allow individual sheep to be sorted into different pens as required. The use of a sorting gate is preferable over 'cutting' with the use of dogs or handlers.

10.2.5   Special Note: Rams, Lambs and Pregnant Ewes; Use of Dogs/Vehicles

Special caution should be taken when working with rams, especially during the mating season. They can become highly aroused by the presence of ewes or other rams and can become aggressive towards handlers. They can attack with sufficient force that they can cause serious leg injuries.

Extra care must be taken when handling or moving pregnant sheep, as any stress can cause significant impact on the female and the unborn foetus; where possible, they should not be handled. Heavily pregnant sheep should preferably not be placed onto their rumps, and particularly not for any long period of time.

During a gather, lambs should be allowed to move at their own pace, as they will tire easily. They should also maintain contact with their dams at all times. Small lambs can become trampled in a holding area, so special caution should taken when gathering and grouping ewes with lambs at foot. Separating off smaller groups at a time may prevent lambs from being trampled. Lambs will also find small gaps in any handling facilities, so

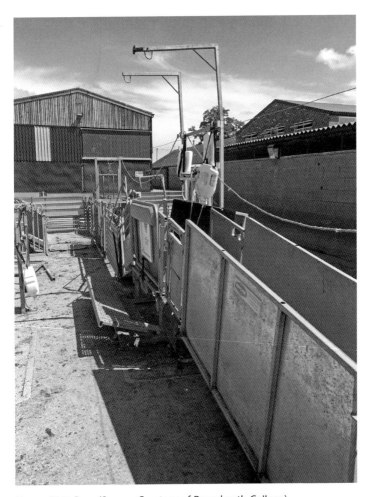

Figure 10.7 Race (Source: Courtesy of Reaseheath College).

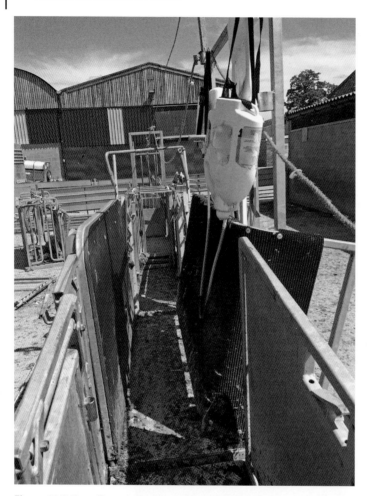

Figure 10.8 Race (Source: Courtesy of Reaseheath College).

they should be designed such that the lamb can escape the area to avoid being trampled but will remain safe if it does so. The lamb will stay nearby to the ewe but may become distressed when they cannot maintain contact with them and vice versa; however, the safety of the lamb and ewe must be a priority.

The use of dogs or humans to drive sheep can be very effective and efficient. However, it is highly stressful for the sheep and, when too much pressure is applied, sheep can stampede, break through fences or try to jump them, thus causing significant damage to themselves and others. Dogs must, therefore, be very carefully controlled and managed if they are to be used. It is unacceptable to allow 'worrying' of sheep by a dog and they must not be allowed to nip or bite the sheep. The positioning and movement of the dog is key to its ability to drive the sheep effectively. A dog should be restrained or removed from an area when sheep are in a small space, so that it does not cause any unnecessary movement or stress to the sheep. If vehicles are to be used, it must be remembered that it is much easier to go faster by vehicle than it is on foot, but the pace of the sheep must be respected.

10.3   How to Approach and Move Goats

10.3.1   Methods and Equipment

Whenever moving or handling goats, the same principles of good preparation as with the sheep are important. Instructions should be clear to all parties, the plans double-checked. Entrances and pathways should be clear of any obstructions and unintended escape routes blocked off.

10.3.2   Moving a Group

Goats are natural followers and it is most preferable to lead goats into a pen rather than to pressure them from the rear. If the goats are used to being handled, the use of some food can encourage them towards the handler due to their inquisitive nature. If a lead doe can be identified, time spent training this goat to come to call or to follow the sound of a feed bucket is time well spent. If the goats are not used to being handled, they may need some encouragement from behind as well as up front with some food. Any pressure from behind should be minimal and the use of dogs is not recommended. Goats, unlike sheep, do not respect dogs; they will turn to face the dog and may attempt to chase the dog away rather than move away from it.

Alternatively, if the space can be made smaller with the use of portable gates, as described for sheep, this may encourage the goats to move forward and into the required area. If goats have kids at foot, sometimes it is easier to catch the kid and allow the nanny goat to follow.

10.3.3   Moving an Individual

Goats should be approached from the side with the handler in clear view of the goat. Approaching slowly and calmly and using the voice to reassure the goat is good practice. Approaching in a friendly manner is a must to maintain a good working relationship with a goat. Most goats will have a collar that can be used to capture and lead it to where it is to be restrained (Figure 10.9).

Goats will also accept being led with the use of a head collar. The head collar must not be allowed to slip down over the nares of the goat, as this will restrict its breathing. If they do not have a collar, the goat can be caught by grasping either a front or rear leg. As soon as the goat has been captured, the hands should be moved, so that one is under the chin and the other placed towards the back end. The hand under the chin will guide the direction of the goat whilst the other hand will encourage it to move forwards (see restraint section for more details). Goats should not be caught or restrained by the horns, as this cause damage to the horns if they are handled incorrectly.

10.3.4   Handling Facilities

Handling facilities for goats should adhere to all the same principles as for sheep, but they must be designed for goats. Goats are generally bigger than sheep, so the facilities

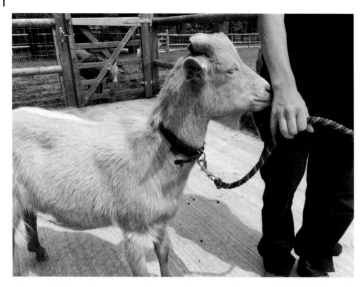

Figure 10.9 Leading a goat (Source: Courtesy of Brinsbury Campus, Chichester College).

must reflect this. Goats that are not used to being handled can jump out of sheep pens as they are very agile, so pens and races should be taller than they are for sheep.

Consideration to the movement of goats through the handling facilities should be given as it is with sheep. Solid walls and curved pens with the use of backing gates can be employed to encourage goats through a race. The floor should be non-slip and the goats should be encouraged forward with the use of a lead doe into a lighter area. Sorting gates can be employed at the end if they are required.

10.3.5   Special Note: Kids, Pregnant Does and Bucks

Bucks, like rams, can be extremely aggressive during the breeding season and extra caution should be taken when in their presence, especially if other bucks or does are present. Bucks can have very large horns that can cause considerable damage to other animals as well as handlers.

Pregnant does should not be subjected to any unnecessary stress and, where possible, heavily pregnant does should not be moved. If any movement through a handling system is required, the facilities should allow for the larger size of the doe through a race without excessive pressure. The doe should be allowed to move at her own pace and careful control of any other goats behind should be managed. Care must be taken when moving pregnant does through any sort of gateway or around corners, so that she does not bang or become squashed against them, potentially damaging the unborn kid.

If does have kids at foot, as with sheep, any movement must be at the pace of the slowest kid and the kid must be allowed to maintain contact with its mother. If groups of does and kids are to be gathered, care must be taken to ensure that kids are not trampled by the adults. Moving smaller groups at a time is better and separating out kids from their does is preferable to maintain their safety.

10.4 How to Restrain a Sheep

10.4.1 Methods and Equipment

When restraining sheep it is important to remember that each individual animal will respond differently. The sheep's temperament, age and previous experience will all have an effect on how it will cope with the restraint. Try to keep restraint to the minimum, using only the required amount needed to get the job done in an efficient and effective manner. Movements should be slow and optimum pressure used.

Some restraint devices are more suitable in certain situations than others and it is important to choose the right method and piece of equipment for the job required. Well-designed facilities should support the animal during restraint and not put any pressure on parts of the body in a manner that may cause injury.

10.4.2 Physical Restraint

The simplest form of restraint for sheep is to hold the animal under the chin with one hand grasping one side of the mandible and the other hand supporting the back end. The sheep can be kept standing and directed easily from this position; wherever the head is pointed, the sheep's body will go. If the animal will not stand still, its body can be held against the side of a pen or wall with the arms and knees. It is preferable to have the rear end of the sheep backed into a corner, unless the recording of rectal temperature or other procedures that require access to this area are being performed. One hand should remain under the chin and one knee placed just in front of the shoulder of the sheep to stop it moving forward; the other knee is placed in the rear flank groove by the hind knee. The remaining hand can be used to either steady the sheep at the back end or to steady the handler against the wall or pen side. Sufficient pressure should be applied to prevent movement but not cause injury.

In open spaces where there is no fence or natural barrier, the sheep can be straddled from behind with the handlers' body as far back as possible over the sheep. One hand should remain under the chin whilst the other reaches as far back as possible to prevent the sheep going backwards. The base of the tail can be held but must not be pulled.

Sheep requiring further restraint or to be restrained for a longer period of time are often tipped or sat on their rump. This is a common method of restraint when access to the feet or udder of the sheep is required. Sheep are usually quiet and easy to handle when placed in this position. Note: heavily pregnant sheep should not be held in this position.

There are a number of ways in which sheep can be placed onto their rumps and the method used will be dictated by the space available and the size of the sheep being tipped. The preferred method (Figures 10.10 to 10.14), if space and strength of the handler allows, is to hold the sheep close to the handler so that it is parallel to the knees.

One hand should be placed under the chin of the sheep and the other hand reaching over the back of the sheep and grasping the flank on the opposite side or placing a hand on or near to this position. The head of the sheep is turned to face the hindquarters and pushed against its shoulder (Figure 10.11).

The handler should at the same time take a step backwards with their leg nearest to the hindquarters and either push the rump or lift the leg using the flank. These actions

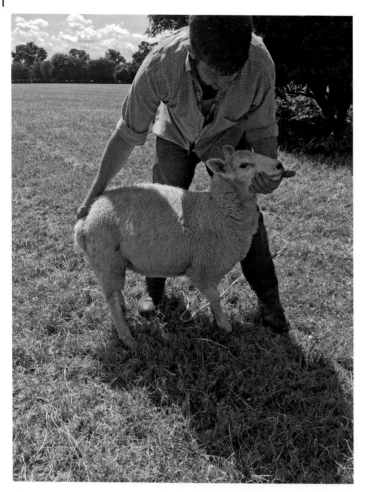

Figure 10.10 Tipping a sheep, Step 1 (Source: Courtesy of Reaseheath College).

should happen simultaneously, so that the sheep is placed off balance and gently slides down the leg (Figures 10.12 and 10.13).

Once the sheep is no longer standing, both hands can be moved to each of the front legs and the sheep moved upwards so that it is sitting on its rump (Figure 10.14). The sheep should be rested on one side of its rump rather than directly on its tail, and its head and back balanced against the legs of the handler. The sheep should be leant slightly backwards at an angle rather than upright to maintain this position.

If the sheep tries to force itself upwards and get to its feet, gentle pressure can be applied to the brisket or breast area to push down gently; this can help to calm it or move it to a more stable position. Alternatively, the sheep's head can be placed to hang gently to the side. This position should only be maintained for a short while to ensure that gases can escape from the rumen to avoid the animal becoming bloated.

Larger sheep can be encouraged to sit on their rump by straddling the sheep and lifting both front legs. Whilst holding the front legs up, the sheep can be encouraged to walk backwards and the handler can then press their knees against the rear legs of the sheep

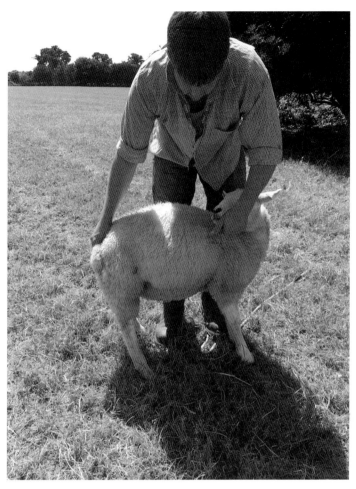

Figure 10.11 Tipping a sheep, Step 2 (Source: Courtesy of Reaseheath College).

lifting it off of its back legs. It should then slowly slide down the handlers' legs until it is on its rump. Alternatively, the sheep can be cradled around its neck with one hand whilst the other hand reaches over to the opposite front leg, which is held up and against the sheep's body. The handler should then push the head and neck backwards to encourage the sheep to walk backwards and trip over the handlers' foot, which is placed behind the back legs. This should lead to the sheep sitting on its rump and it can then be straightened into the correct position.

It may take two people to place large sheep or rams onto their rump. In this case, each person should hold either the two front legs or the two hind legs, with the body resting against the legs of the handlers. Simultaneously, both handlers should lift the legs and allow the sheep to slide down the legs of the handler so that the sheep is sitting on its side. Each person can help to lift the front end so that it is lifted to sit on its rump.

If the sheep needs to be restrained for a longer period, specially designed equipment such as neck yokes, squeeze chutes or clamps should be used. A sheep can be stood in a neck yoke for a period of time or, if it will accept it, tied up with a halter. Halters must be

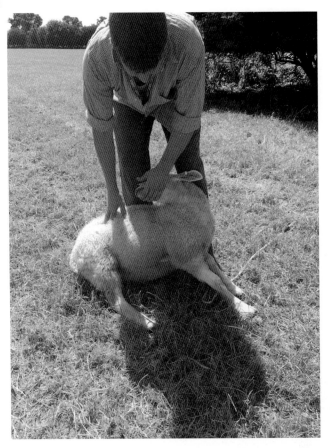

Figure 10.12 Tipping a sheep, Step 3 (Source: Courtesy of Reaseheath College).

fitted correctly such that they do not drop over and obstruct the nares of the sheep. Squeeze cutes or clamps can hold a sheep in position for a reasonable amount of time and allow the handler the freedom to move around the sheep and perform all necessary tasks. Other equipment, such as turning tables or chairs that allow the operator to have both hands free to carry out work, are commercially available. Care should be taken when using such equipment that the correct pressure is applied for each animal to avoid any unnecessary stress or injury to it.

More aversive methods of restraint are available if they are required. These can include the use of ropes or a gambrel. A gambrel is a curved device that fits over the neck of a sheep lying on its chest; its forefeet are individually lifted onto crooks on top of the gambrel. The legs push down on the gambrel; this exerts force on the neck to keep the sheep grounded. Ropes can also be used to keep a sheep lying on the ground if required. A large circular piece of rope should be placed around the lower legs of the sheep, just above the hock, while the sheep is sitting on its rump. The section of rope behind the sheep's legs is pulled upwards between the legs, so creating two small loops around the hind legs, and is then placed over the back of the sheep's neck. The sheep should then be laid on the ground onto its sternum.

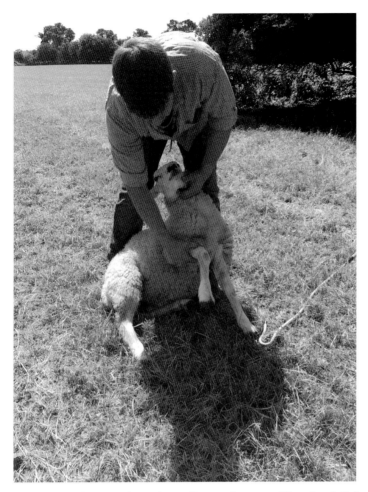

Figure 10.13 Tipping a sheep, Step 4 (Source: Courtesy of Reaseheath College).

Sometimes, there are procedures that you will need to carry out on your own. The sheep can be restrained by straddling it and backing it into a corner so that it cannot move backwards. Place the head behind your elbow and use this to lift the head from under the chin upwards and backwards, moving it away from your body towards the wall.

If lambs need to be restrained, they can be held by their front legs in one hand with your other hand holding the body of the lamb against your own body. The lamb's body can be rested on the raised knee of the handler and the front feet allowed to hang down, leaving the hands free for any treatment or observations required. Alternatively, the lamb can be cradled with one arm slid under the sternum of the lamb so that the legs are free to hang either side. To restrain a lamb for castration, the two legs from each side should be held in each hand with the back pressed against the chest of the handler or, if performing the castration on your own, sit the lamb on your lap so that

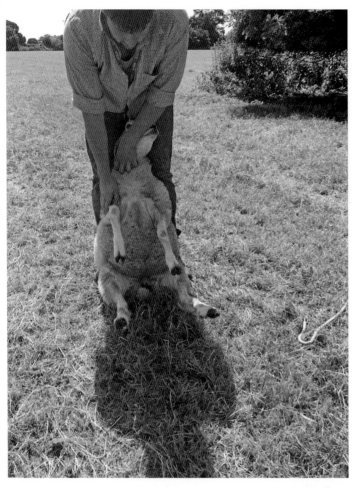

Figure 10.14 Tipping a sheep, Step 5 (Source: Courtesy of Reaseheath College).

the scrotum and tail are exposed using one forearm across the lambs chest to hold it in place.

10.4.3   Training for Restraint

Sheep can be trained from an early age to accept the halter and accept restraint (Figures 10.15 and 10.16). The earlier handling and training can begin, the easier sheep will be to handle.

Lambs handled early enough in a friendly manner will build a better relationship with their handlers and this can lead to a bond being formed. Bonded sheep are more likely to approach their handler, reducing the need for pressure to be applied when gathering or when handling. Sheep can even be trained to enter a race and even enter a restraint, such as a tilt table or clamp, with the use of positive reinforcement, such as receiving a food reward at the restraint. Even after aversive treatment, sheep can be retrained to accept the restraint (Grandin, 1989).

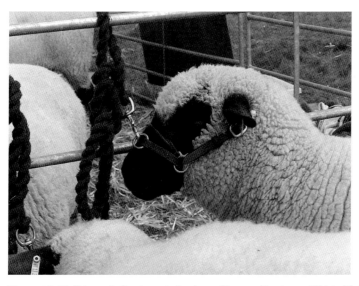

Figure 10.15 Using a halter to restrain sheep (Source: Courtesy of Krista McLennan, 2016).

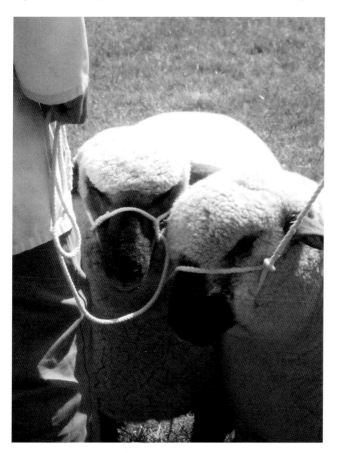

Figure 10.16 Using a halter to restrain sheep (Source: Courtesy of Krista McLennan, 2016).

10.5 How to Restrain Goats

10.5.1 Methods and Equipment

When restraining goats, as with the sheep, an individual's temperament, age and previous experience will impact upon how it copes with being restrained. The methods used to restrain a goat are quite similar to those used in sheep. However, goats can be more difficult to handle compared to sheep due to their agility and strength. Goats have the ability to stand up on their hind legs and jump forward, making them dangerous to handle. The use of the minimum amount of restraint required is encouraged, as goats can become stressed more easily than sheep when handling, and will lie down in learned helplessness. Precaution must be made to restrain goats in a manner that decreases their stress levels but is safe for all parties involved and there are varying restraint devices available, each having a different level of pressure or averseness to the goat. It is important to choose the right method and piece of equipment for the job required.

10.5.2 Physical Restraint

Once a goat has been caught, either by the collar or by grasping a front or back leg, the handler should move their hands to restrain the goat in a more effective and safe manner. One hand should be placed either under the chin of the goat elevating the head slightly (Figure 10.17) or around the chest of the goat, whilst the other hand can be placed towards the back end of the goat to steady it and prevent it from moving backwards. ***The tail should never be pulled to restrain the goat***.

If the goat has a collar (Figure 10.18) sometimes it is only necessary to hold this to prevent the goat moving away. Goats can easily be restrained by the use of a halter if they have been trained to accept one. Make sure the halter does not slip down the nose and constrict the nares.

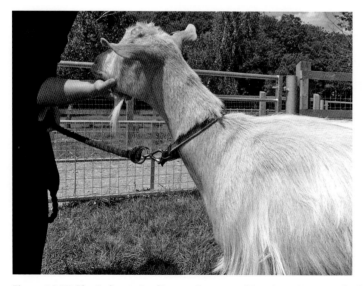

Figure 10.17 Physical restraint (Source: Courtesy of Brinsbury Campus, Chichester College).

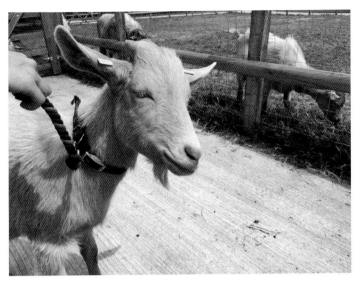

Figure 10.18 Use of a collar and lead (Source: Courtesy of Brinsbury Campus, Chichester College).

If further restraint of the head is required, one hand should be placed under the chin whilst the other hand encircles the back of the head. Alternatively, the handler can straddle the goat and place a hand on either side of the head, with the fingers wrapped around the mandible holding it firmly. If working on the goat alone, goats can be straddled and backed into a corner, with one hand under the chin and lifting to control the head, leaving the other hand free to carry out any husbandry required. Precautions should be taken in any of the positions if the animal has horns, especially when trying to control the head from behind (Figure 10.19).

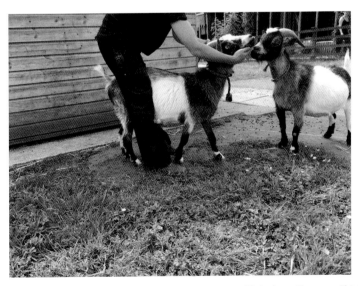

Figure 10.19 Physical restraint (Source: Courtesy of Brinsbury Campus, Chichester College).

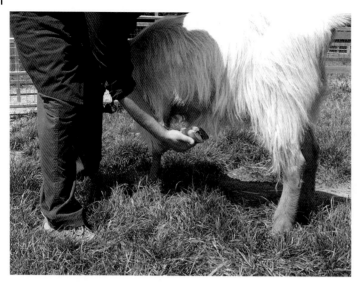

Figure 10.20 Holding up a front leg for additional restraint (Source: Courtesy of Brinsbury Campus, Chichester College).

If the goat will not stand, either a front leg can be held up against the body (Figure 10.20) or the goat can be moved up against a wall (Figures 10.21 and 10.22) and pressure applied with one knees in the flank area and a hand by the collar or neck, or both knees can be used to apply pressure as described in the sheep section.

If it is possible, backing the goat into a corner can help to prevent it from moving backwards, leaving the handler just to prevent the animal from moving forward by controlling the head. As with sheep, if the handler can control the head by holding the chin, the goat can be directed or held in position.

If the goat needs to be worked on for a longer period of time or access is needed to its abdomen, the goat can be placed onto its side. *The goat must not be placed onto its rump like sheep*, as it does not have enough padding to protect its bones and this can cause bruising.

To place the goat onto its side, the goat should be stood parallel to the handlers' legs. Using similar principles as with sheep, the goat should be placed off balance by turning the head to face the rump by grasping under the chin and nose with a hand, whilst the other hand reaches over the back of the goat and grabs the near rear leg pulling it forward. The goat should then fall backwards and down the handler's leg onto its side. Alternatively, the handler should reach over the goats back with both arms. One hand should grasp the flank at the rear of the goat and the other hand should grasp the near fore leg just above the knee. Simultaneously both the leg and flank should be lifted so that the goats' legs are lifted off the ground and the goat placed gently onto its side. The arm and elbow at the front of the goat should be used to control the head and neck of the goat. To prevent the goat from rising, a knee can be gently placed onto the neck of the goat and the hands placed firmly on the legs to prevent them from moving.

If available, equipment such as a milking or foot trimming stanchion can be used to restrain the head of the goat. Some facilities may also contain a headgate or roll table that can allow the head of the goat or its entire body to be held. Roll tables can be used to gain

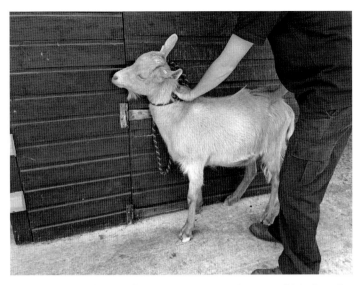

Figure 10.21 Further standing restraint (Source: Courtesy of Brinsbury Campus, Chichester College).

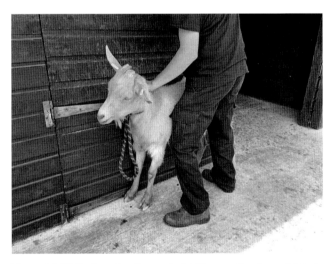

Figure 10.22 Further standing restraint (Source: Courtesy of Brinsbury Campus, Chichester College).

access to goat's feet for trimming. However, these can be aversive to the goat and special care should be taken when using this type of equipment on goats that may not be used to this type of restraint.

If restraining buck goats, special care must be taken. They can be particularly dangerous during mating season and can take out the legs of handler with a single head butt. They are incredibly strong and should be respected. Due to their size and strength they may need fiercer handling, but this should not be aversive. Each buck will need different restraint pressures and the method used should be designed for that goat.

Goat kids should be caught by the body and not the legs as this can cause dislocation. The goat kid should be held so that one arm is placed under the length of the sternum and its legs allowed to hang down freely, either side of the handlers' arms. If carrying more than one kid at a time, each kid should be tucked under the arm by placing the arm under the chest area with the legs free to hang down. To restrain a kid, hold it against your body with one hand holding the head and neck area, whilst the other hand is free to carry out any tasks required.

10.5.3   Training for Restraint

Goats are fairly easy to train for handling and restraint due to their inquisitive and friendly nature. They are willing to work a relationship with their handler. Early, friendly handling of kids is key. Good quality early life experience leads to a better human–animal relationships, which, in turn, make the kids easier to handle.

Adult goats that experience gentling will become habituated to human presence and will be more willing to approach a human compared to goats that have not received any previous handling (Jackson and Hackett, 2007). Goats can be trained in a similar manner to sheep with positive reinforcement techniques through the use of positive food rewards. They can be trained to accept the collar, a halter or even the turntable. Taking the time to train a goat goes a long way to reducing stress during handling for both the goat and the handler.

10.6   Special Considerations

Sheep and goats can become difficult to handle if forced to do anything that is unnatural to them. Patience is important. Early, friendly handling is key.

Key Points

- Sheep and goats must be handled differently according to their natural behavioural strengths.
- Use the flight zone and point of balance to move a group of sheep.
- Keep sheep together as a group.
- A calm flock of sheep is much easier to move.
- Work in dry, cool conditions as much as possible, especially when moving sheep.
- A sheep can be trained to be the 'leader' of the group.
- Stay calm, gentle handling is more effective than force.
- Sheep should not be held on their sides, backs or rumps for more than a few minutes if their rumen is full or if they are heavily pregnant.
- Goats should not be sat on their rumps, as they have less padding in this area and it could cause serious damage.
- Electric goads are ineffective in sheep and should not be used.
- Wool, ears, tail, legs and horns should not be pulled or used for physical restraint. The only time horns should be held is for the safety of the person restraining the sheep or goat. Other methods of restraint should also be employed in this situation.

- Minimize isolation of sheep and goats.
- Slower is faster.

Self-assessment Questions

1 Describe the process you would use to move a group of sheep.

2 Rather than 'cut' an individual or small group from the rest of the flock, what is a better way to separate an individual for examination?

3 What are the key considerations when gathering sheep off a hill?

4 What is the difference between sheep and goats in terms of flocking instinct and how does this affect the way a group is moved?

5 Goats should never be placed on their rumps. Explain why.

6 Name three similar ways you can restrain a goat or sheep.

Answers can be found in the back of the book.

References

Boivin, X. and Braastad, B.O. (1996) Effects of handling during temporary isolation after early weaning on goat kids' later response to humans. *Applied Animal Behaviour Science*, **48**, 61–71.

Boivin, X., Tournadre, H. and Le Neindre, P. (2000) Hand-feeding and gentling influence early-weaned lambs' attachment responses to their stockperson. *Journal of Animal Science*, **78**, 879–884.

Bremner, K.J., Braggins, J. B. and Kilgour, R., (1980) Training sheep as 'leaders' in abattoirs and farm sheep yards. *Proceedings of the New Zealand Society of Animal Production*, **40**, 111–116.

Grandin, T. (1989) Voluntary acceptance of restraint by sheep. *Applied Animal Behaviour Science*, **23**, 257–261.

Guesgen, M.J., Beausoleil, N.J. and Stewart, M. (2013) Effects of early human handling in the pain sensitivity of young lambs. *Veterinary Anaesthesia and Analgesia*, **40**, 55–62.

Hiendleder, S., Kaupe, B., Wassmuth, R. and Janke, A. (2002) Molecular analysis of wild and domestic sheep questions current nomenclature and provides evidence for domestication from two different subspecies. *Proceedings of the Royal Society London B*, **269**, 893–904.

Jackson, K.M.A. and Hackett, D. (2007) A note: The effects of human handling on heart girth, behaviour and milk quality in dairy goats. *Applied Animal Behaviour Science*, **108**, 332–336.

Luikart, G., Gielly, L., Excoffier, L. *et al.* (2001) Multiple maternal origins and weak phylogeographic structure in domestic goats. *Proceedings of the National Academy of Sciences of the USA*, **98** (10), 5927–5932.

Markowitz, T.M., Dally, M.R., Gursky, K. and Price, E.O. (1998) Early handling increases lamb affinity for humans. *Animal Behaviour*, **55**, 573–587.

Further Reading

Grandin, T. (ed) (2015) *Improving Animal Welfare. A Practical Approach*, 2nd edn, CABI (Centre for Agriculture and Biosciences International), Wallingford, UK.
Sheldon, C.C., Sonsthagen, T. and Topel, J.A. (2006) *Animal Restraint for Veterinary Professionals*, Mosby, Maryland Heights, MO.

11

Handling and Restraint of Pigs

Krista M. McLennan[1] and Stella J. Chapman[2]

[1]*Chester University, Chester, UK*
[2]*University Centre Hartpury, Gloucestershire, UK*

As with many of the domesticated farm animal species, the exact timeline of domestication events in pigs is controversial. The modern agricultural pig that we see on farms today is descended from the European wild boar (*Sus scrofa*), a member of the family Suidae, which is a group of pig species that originated some 20–30 million years ago from the order of Certartiodactyla (Frantz *et al.*, 2016). Whilst many of the physical and productive characteristics have changed, their behavioural instincts have been largely conserved (Edwards, 2011). Domestication is believed to have occurred first in the Near East approximately 9000 years ago; however, it is yet to be established whether domesticated pigs that show a marked morphological difference with their wild ancestors have a single or multiple origin (Giuffra *et al.*, 2000). Domestication of a species is, in part, a geographical event and this has been demonstrated in the pig with two separate domestication events being recognized in southwest Asia (now known as Turkey) and in China.

Farmed pigs are found in almost all regions of the world and supply approximately 40% of the world meat supply, although eating of pork is restricted within the religious views of Moslems and Jews (Edwards, 2011). Pigs are also kept as part of animal collections and there has been a growing trend in recent years to keep them as pets, particularly the miniature pigs that are being bred. It is important to remember, however, that in many countries any pig that is kept is regarded as a farm animal, and thus falls under the specific legislation for that animal.

11.1 Behaviour

Pigs are highly gregarious and live in groups of approximately 15–20 individuals consisting of mothers and their offspring. Male pigs or boars are often on their own or in small bachelor groups until mating time. The group has a strong hierarchy with one individual dominant over the rest. This can make them aggressive if not mixed with other animals. Pigs would naturally spend the majority of their time foraging as a group with their snouts searching through their environments for food. This makes them highly inquisitive by nature.

Safe Handling and Restraint of Animals: A Comprehensive Guide, First Edition. Stella J. Chapman.
© 2018 John Wiley & Sons Ltd. Published 2018 by John Wiley & Sons Ltd.

The pig is a prey species and thus will have a natural tendency to flee from a dangerous situation before it will fight. This means that the pig will prefer to escape and can fit through small spaces if needed. This can also make pigs quite dangerous, as due to their size and strength they will try to push past or run through people if they can see a gap. If they are unable to flee, their primary form of defence is their teeth. A pig may try to chase and bite a person if they feel threatened.

Pigs, unlike the other prey species, have their eyes on the front of their face. They have still retained a panoramic view of their environment with a blind spot at the rear, but their eyesight is very poor. They rely mostly on their good sense of smell and excellent sense of hearing. They do have an individual flight zone and their point of balance remains at the shoulder.

11.1.1   How this Can Affect Handling

Pigs can be very difficult to handle and restrain due to their large size and strong nature. Their slim line body shape and strength means that holding the pig by hand is too difficult and too dangerous. Pure physical strength will be no match for a large pig. Their poor eyesight can make them very fearful, as they cannot see where they are going very well, so may be reluctant to enter a new area without proper inspection. If they are fearful of an environment or situation and are thus feeling threatened, this could lead a pig to become aggressive. Rough handling will increase the chances of the pig slipping, falling or turning around to face the handler (Rabaste *et al.*, 2007). They have very sharp teeth and can do a lot of damage to a person. Pigs cannot sweat, so can overheat quickly if they become too stressed. Any method of handling or restraint must be quick and effective to avoid stress and injury to the pig and handler.

Due to their poor depth perception, they can bauk at simple distractions, such as changes of floor type, or changes in light, such as shadows. Pigs can also be easily startled due to their poor eyesight, so you must make sure that the pig is aware of your presence at all time. Pigs also do not like to move into the darkness, to move up or down steep ramps, or around tight turns. This must be considered when moving them around and during handling and restraint.

Pigs, due to their strong grouping instinct, want to maintain visual if not body contact with another pig. Isolation is very stressful to a pig, so they must be kept together. Despite having a strong grouping instinct, they cannot be herded in the same manner as ruminant species.

11.1.2   How to Use Behavioural Traits to Effect When Handling

It is important when handling pigs that tasks are carried out in a slow and steady manner. The handler must move in a slow and deliberate manner and should use their voice as much as possible, so that the pig is aware of where the handler is at all times. Talking to the pig in a reassuring manner will keep the pig calm throughout the process and make handling much easier. The pig must be allowed to walk at its own pace and must be allowed time to inspect its environment. Do not force a pig, but encourage it into an area.

Moving pigs in groups of three or four will make handling and moving of pigs much easier. This is especially so when one individual may need treating; moving two or three together will reduce the stress experienced and make the job easier and quicker to carry out.

When moving pigs, the use of a lead animal is beneficial, as pigs will follow the animal in front of them. This is so they maintain contact with the group or individual. Using the same principles of pressure and release as outlined in the cattle and small ruminants' chapter, the pig can be encouraged forward by entering into its flight zone. Once the animal moves forward, pressure is released by the stepping out of the flight zone. Pressure can be reapplied by the handler by continuing to enter the space around the individual. It is important that this is carried out in a slow and deliberate manner to give the pig time to move forward. The handler can position themselves around the point of balance at the shoulder of the pig to move them forwards or backwards. Due to the poor eyesight of pigs, the use of a board or solid walls is encouraged to guide the direction of the pig, as they will move away from a solid form.

On farms, pigs can be housed in a number of ways and this should be considered when planning any handling or restraint. For example, groups of pigs can be housed inside large barns on straw (Figure 11.1), or they may be in large open fields.

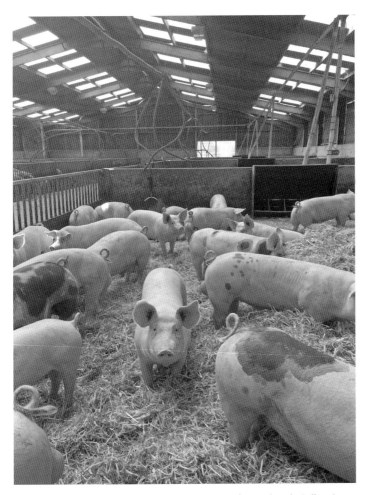

Figure 11.1 Housing of pigs (Source: Courtesy of Reaseheath College).

For mothers with their piglets, it is important that they have a separate space away from the rest of the group. This allows mother and offspring to bond without the added concern of other group members. In Figure 11.2 it can be seen that there is a separate area for sleeping, with a straw bed and area where the piglets and mother can come outside onto a concreted area. Figure 11.3 shows that within the pen the feeding station is set up so that the sow can be restrained in this area. Taking note of these types of facilities can help with any planning.

It should be noted that any facilities that are being used for handling should have non-slip flooring and, as pigs can become easily distracted, solid sided curved chutes should be used where possible if moving a large group. Keeping areas well lit and free from significantly contrasting light will allow the pig to move forward easily. This all helps to remove any unnecessary stress for the pig, leading to calmer animals that can be handled safely and effectively. Keeping animals under some form of shelter and out of the elements is a must, particularly in hot weather, due to the pigs' inability to sweat.

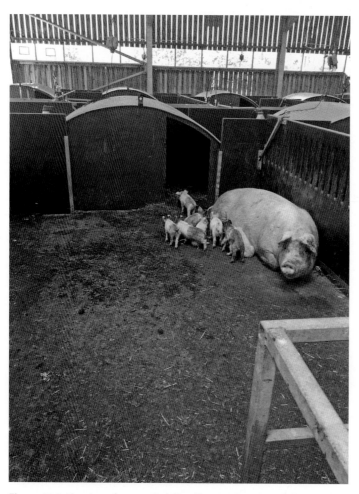

Figure 11.2 Housing of sow and piglets (Source: Courtesy of Reaseheath College).

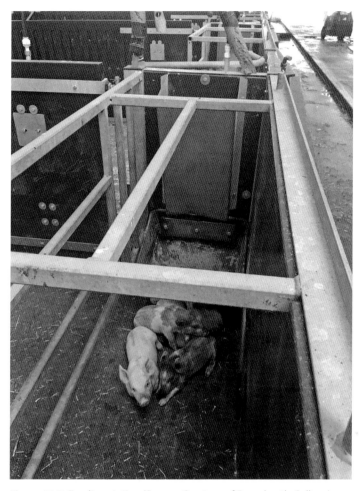

Figure 11.3 Feeding station (Source: Courtesy of Reaseheath College).

11.2 How to Approach and Move Pigs

11.2.1 General Methods and Equipment

When moving pigs, as with all other animals it is important to ensure that plans have been made as to where they are to be moved and how. Each member of the team should know what they are required to do. Make sure that all corridors are free from obstruction and that all escape routes for the pig are sealed off. The way in which the pig or pigs are to walk should be obvious and should be well lit with no shadows or sudden change in lighting. This is to help prevent the pig(s) from bauking or having to spend too much time investigating. Pigs should be moved from darker to lighter areas if there is a contrast and it is recommended that floors should be even and not slope, as this can cause leg injuries (DEFRA, 2003). There should be no tight turns but a curved area provided that will allow the pig to maintain visual contact with the one in front. It is important that when working with pigs there is an escape route available for the handler should the pig become aggressive.

Good handling comes from treating the pig in a humane manner. Pigs that are handled well will not be fearful or apprehensive about being handled or moved, and are thus unlikely to look for an escape route. A good human–animal relationship should be established early on, as it is vital for effective and humane handling of pigs. This can be formed through gently touching the pig and talking to it in a calm manner, as well as feeding it in the close vicinity of a human to help to train the animal that handling is a positive experience. It is often best to ask the person who knows the pig best to approach and handle the pig.

Whenever approaching swine it is important to make your presence known to them by using your voice so as not to startle them. Your approach should be slow and steady. Pigs that are used to being handled may well come towards the handler to investigate when they are aware of their presence.

The use of pig boards (various sizes for different jobs), paddles, wooden sticks, noise shakers and stock flags can be used to encourage the pig(s) forward (Figures 11.4 and 11.5).

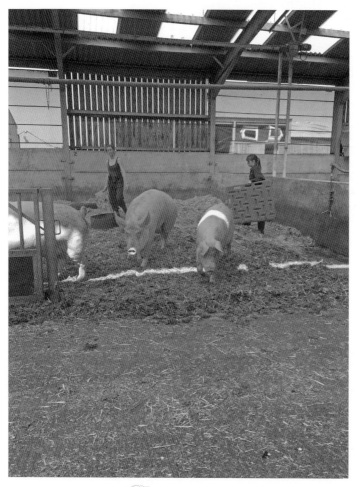

Figure 11.4 Use of boards to move pigs (Source: Courtesy of Reaseheath College).

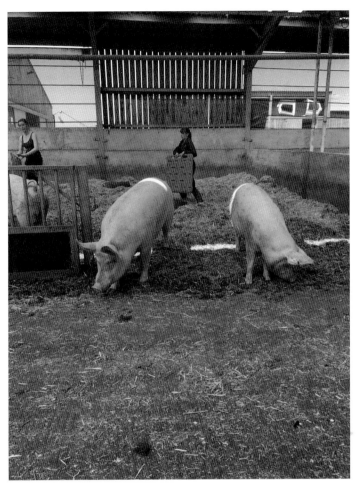

Figure 11.5 Use of boards to move pigs (Source: Courtesy of Reaseheath College).

They should only be used as an extension to the arm and should never be used to hit or smack an animal. A pig should only be encouraged to move forward if the way ahead is clear and they should be allowed to do so at their own pace. Avoid making too much noise or force that may increase the arousal of the animal. Keeping the pig(s) calm will make for easier handling in the long run. Excessive force should not be required to move a pig in anyway.

11.2.2 Moving a Group of Pigs

It is best to move pigs in a small group of three or four (Figure 11.6).

Moving large groups increases the stress experienced by pigs (Lewis and McGlone, 2007) and it will be hard to move the group in a calm manner. A large board can be used to separate off a small group of pigs from a larger group; the smaller group can

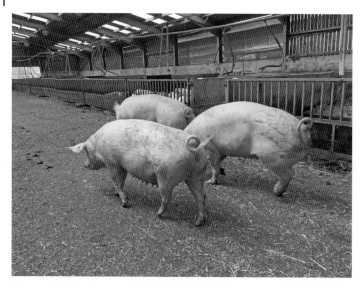

Figure 11.6 Moving a small group of sows (Source: Courtesy of Reaseheath College).

then be guided out into an area such as a corridor or race. This board can be used to block off an area where the pigs need to move away from, as well as direct the pig into a space by setting it against or to the side of the pig. Using the principles of the point of balance, if the board is in front of the pigs head, the pig will go backwards. If the pig can see a clear path in front of it and the board allows the pig to go forward, it moves forwards.

If pressure from the board is used to direct the head in the opposite direction from the handler, the pig will turn away from the board. If the board is opened up, the pig will move towards the board. Flags and noise shakers can be used to encourage the pigs forward without the need for touching the animal and can be used from behind the group, as they encourage the whole group to move forward, not just the pigs at the rear. If further encouragement is needed, paddles and wooden sticks can be used to tap the lead pig on the shoulder to encourage it to move forward. Once the lead pig moves, the rest of the group should continue forward. Paddles, sticks or other items used to encourage the pigs forward should never be used to hit or smack the pig.

It is important when moving a group of pigs that you keep the group together and do not let the group break away. This is done by ensuring that the direction of travel is clear and that the pigs cannot escape through small gaps (Figures 11.7 and 11.8).

Keeping the pigs calm and moving them slowly will allow the lead pig to inspect the area and prevent the pigs from becoming fearful of the situation and looking for an escape route. Do not continue to push the other pigs from behind if the lead pig is not moving forward. Wait until the lead pig has started to move again before reapplying pressure. Once the pigs are in the place required, the large board can be used to reduce any space and restrict the pig's movement, holding them in the required area.

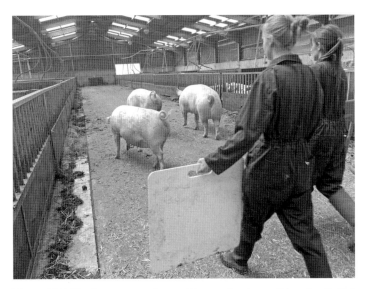

Figure 11.7 Moving a group of sows (Source: Courtesy of Reaseheath College).

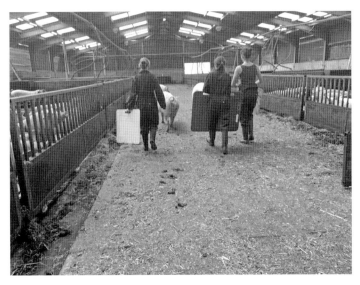

Figure 11.8 Moving a group of sows (Source: Courtesy of Reaseheath College).

11.2.3 Moving the Individual

It is difficult to capture just one pig out of a group. It is best to take a small group of three or four and separate them out from the rest of the group, as described above. Once a small group has been held in an area, an individual pig can be penned off in this area or restrained in a manner that will allow them to maintain visual contact with the other animals. This will reduce the stress levels experienced by the pigs and will make handling easier. Boards or solid hurdles (flat solid objects used to protect the legs of the handler) can be used to separate and direct a pig away from the group into a small handling pen. The board must be solid so that the pig cannot see through it, as they will see this as an escape route.

Items such as paddles, sticks, the brush from a broom or flags can also be used to encourage the pig to go forward or can be used to help separate out one pig from a small group. Gently tap the pig on the shoulder or side of the face to encourage it to move away from the paddle or stick and continue to move forward. If the pig moves in the wrong direction, to prevent any further forward movement use a hurdle or the flag to stop the pig rather than tapping the pig on the nose with the stick. Again, the paddles and sticks must never be used to hit or slap the animal. This can cause pain and bruising as well as potentially enraging the pig and causing it to become aggressive towards the handler. It may be necessary to cover the pigs' eyes in order to encourage it to walk backwards, away from the cover. An item such as a bucket can be placed gently over the snout and head of the pig. They will walk backwards away from the cover. This can be used to help guide the pig into an area in a calm manner. It should be removed as soon as the pig is held in place with a board or is contained in some other manner. Small pressure applied to the tail by lifting it slightly upwards and forwards can help to direct the pig into position. It must not be pushed excessively or twisted, as this is highly aversive and can be painful.

If a pig is small enough, two people may be able to lift it to move it. The pig should be lifted by placing it on its side and the body of the pig placed against the bodies of the handlers. One person should put one arm around the front end of the pig by placing an arm underneath the chest area and the other arm over the top of the pigs' body, interlocking their arms around the pig. The other person should do the same at the rear end but placing their arms around the flank area. Keeping the pig on its side to prevent it from wriggling free can help to keep the animal calm. Minimal pressure pushing the pigs' body towards that of the handlers will help to keep the pig safe and feel calm whilst being moved. Pigs should not be placed on their backs and should never be held by their legs, upside down.

11.2.4   Sows, Boars, Finishers and Piglets

Piglets can be moved by grabbing a back leg and lifting them by placing a hand under the chest and another under their flank to help support their body. The hand under the flank can be moved and placed over the top of the piglet to keep them calm. The piglet should be held against the chest of the handler to make it feel secure (Figure 11.9).

If two piglets are to be moved, the piglets' body can be supported by the forearm and hand of the handler with their legs hanging down either side and the body held against that of the handler as before.

To place the piglet down, its front legs must be placed on the ground first and then the rest of its body (Figure 11.10).

Piglets must never be lifted by their ears or by their front legs.

Sows, especially those who have piglets at foot, can be very aggressive, as they have very strong mothering instincts. Piglets when handled can squeal very loudly to warn the mother that they are being handled. Be very careful when handling piglets with a sow nearby. Large male pigs or boars can also be very aggressive. When handling them they should be penned separately, so that they do not cause damage to other

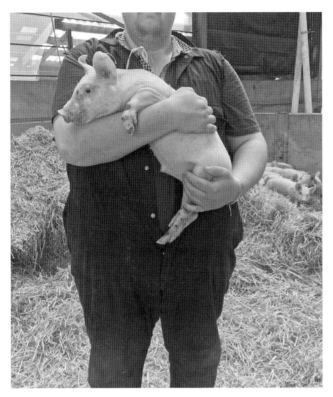

Figure 11.9 Restraint of a piglet (Source: Courtesy of Reaseheath College).

pigs, but they should still be able to make contact with or be within visual range of other pigs.

11.3 How to Restrain Pigs

11.3.1 Methods and Equipment

Before restraining a pig make sure that all necessary equipment is to hand and that any procedure has been carefully planned so that it can be carried out quickly. This will reduce any unnecessary stress to the animal. Any restraint used should be as much as is required to allow the job to be carried out safely and quickly. Minimal use of restraint for as short amount of time as far as is possible, is better for the pigs' welfare and for the handler in the long term.

Most pigs can be restrained simply by restricting the size of the area they are in and removing their ability to move forward by blocking the head and body with a pig board. Some pigs may be restrained simply by providing them with some food. This will depend on their previous experience.

It is important when restraining pigs that they are kept as calm and as stress-free as possible. This will keep the pig still throughout the procedure and help to ensure high standards of good welfare are maintained. This can be achieved by keeping a firm hand on the pig and using a soft low tone of voice in a calm manner.

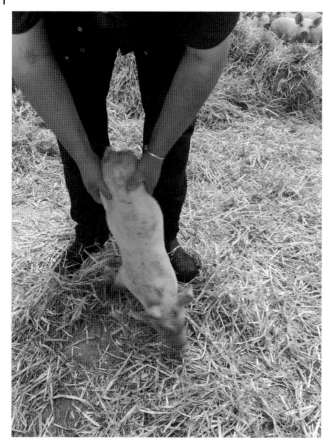

Figure 11.10 Releasing a piglet back to the ground following restraint (Source: Courtesy of Reaseheath College).

11.3.2 Physical Restraint

Boards or hurdles can be used for restraining pigs in different ways depending on the individual pig and the procedure that is required. Boards can be used to restrict the pig from moving forwards or backwards, and large boards can be used by two people to hold a pig in an area or to apply pressure against the pig when up near a wall. With smaller pigs and where the board may be small, the handler can place their leg into the flank area and hindquarters to help secure the pig against a flat surface. When restraining a pig in this manner it is best to try and make a 'V' shape with the board or hurdle and place the pigs head in the smaller section of the 'V' and then use either a board or your knees to hold the pig in place.

If further restraint is required and if facilities are available, the following equipment should be used to help control a pig. **Weigh crates** or **trapping crates** may be used (Figure 11.11) to help restrain larger pigs and if they need to be restrained for a longer period of time than is possible by usinng boards. Pigs should be funnelled slowly into a crate from an area where they are being held through the use of boards, as described in Section 11.2.

For small-to-medium-sized pigs, a **sling** can be used to help restrain the pig by lifting it gently and very slightly off the ground. Pigs can be trained to walk onto the sling and

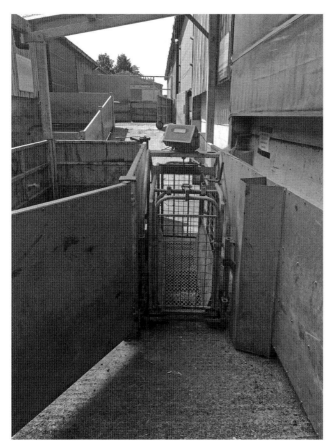

Figure 11.11 Restraint crate (Source: Courtesy of Reaseheath College).

place each of their feet into the required holes, so that the sling can be wrapped around the pig's body with all four limbs held straight down. A sling can be adjusted to take a number of sized pigs and, if trained, can be a stress free and minimal restraint method that keeps the pig and handler safe.

Small pigs or piglets can be placed into a small 'V'-shaped **trough**, so that they can be placed on their back. The pig's front legs should be held down towards its body with one hand whilst the other hand holds the pig's head, gently pushing it backwards. A rope can also be tied around the back legs of the pig to help leave the hands free to perform other procedures or provide support to the pig. This method should only be used when necessary, for the minimum time necessary, as it can be very stressful to the pig or piglet.

If a pig cannot be moved but still needs to be restrained, the pig can be **cast,** or placed on its side. If the pig is small enough, the handler(s) should stand parallel to the pig with the body against their legs. The handler should reach over the top of the pig's body and grasp the near fore and hind legs, pulling the pig off balance and allowing it to fall to the side. If there are two people available, each person can grasp both of the front or rear legs and pull the pig so that it falls gently to the side. Where the pig may be too large for this, ropes may be required. Attach a rope to the front and rear foot of the same side of the pig, pass the rope under the pig's abdomen and pull it up and over the top of the pig, so that its feet are dislodged from underneath its body causing it to fall to the side. After each of these procedures, when the pig is on its side, pressure should be applied by the handler(s) using their knees on the flank and shoulder area, holding down the legs of the pig so that it cannot get upright again.

Piglets or very small pigs can be restrained by holding them by their back legs and placing their bodies between the knees of the handler such that their front feet still touch the ground in front. The knees are used to apply the right amount of pressure that is required to prevent the pig from moving free.

Piglets and other smaller pigs can be held by the stockperson for restraint. They should be picked up by placing one hand under the chest area, using the other hand to support the piglet under the flank. The piglet should be held close to the handler's chest with one arm coming up underneath the front legs and the hand laid over the back of the pig's neck. The other hand should hold both rear legs against the chest of the handler. Piglets can be captured by grasping one or both back legs. Although they can be picked up by their back legs and held in this manner, it is not the preferred option and they should be picked up by the method as previously described. If castrating or tail docking piglets it may be necessary to expose the pigs' rear end. The piglet can be placed between the handlers legs so that its rear end is facing out, with the body allowed to hang down behind the handler. The handler can then use both hands to hold the legs apart, exposing the scrotum area ready for surgery.

The use of a **hog snare** or **snubbing rope** should only be used when all other restraint methods cannot be used for whatever reason, as they are highly stressful to the pig and can cause significant damage if not used correctly. A hog snare can be made from a number of materials, such as plastic, wood or metal with rope at the end. The snare consists of a piece of piping for the handle with a piece of string looped at the end of the handle; the string can be pulled tight once over the nose of the pig. To restrain a pig using a snare, the loop of rope should be placed in front of the pig's snout to encourage the pig to investigate it with its mouth. Once the piece of string is within the pigs' mouth, the string should be pulled gently upwards so that a loop is created over the top of the nose. The string should at the same time also be placed as far back in the mouth as possible, behind the tusks and close to the commissure of the mouth before it is tightened. When the rope is tightened over the pigs' snout, the pig will react aversively and may squeal very loudly whilst pulling away from the pressure around its mouth. Perform any procedure required as quickly as possible and release the pig when safe to do so by pushing down on the handle loosening the string and moving the string away from the pig's mouth. The snare should only be placed for a few minutes and pigs should never be moved by a snare or tied to anything whilst using the snare. The use of wire should never be used as this can cause damage to the pigs' snout.

11.3.3 Training for Restraint

Pigs are highly intelligent animals and can be easily trained for both movement and restraint. The stress experience for the pig can be reduced with even minimal training (Lewis *et al.*, 2008). Older, well trained animals can be used as a guide for younger more naïve pigs. Pigs are very much a creature of habit and they like to maintain a routine. This can be used throughout the training period by getting them used to a certain procedure or piece of equipment as part of their normal daily routine. Moving them on a regular basis will mean that it will be part of the routine for the pig.

Training begins with building a good human–animal relationship. Pigs are highly intelligent and respond very well to voice and gentling procedures. Stockpersons who speak regularly to their pigs in a calm voice and gently place a firm and comforting hand on the animal find it goes a long way towards training pigs and getting them used to human contact. Building up a trust partnership is key; the use of food is also a good way of training pigs.

11.4 Special Considerations

- Pigs overheat quickly if they are handled too roughly for long periods.
- Pigs are prone to high levels of stress and fear, leading to exhaustion, overheating and even death.
- Piglets are fragile and should be handled with care.
- Bones are easily broken if pulled or grasped incorrectly.
- Incorrectly handled pigs will become fearful and aggressive.
- Special considerations should be given to handling boars, or sows when they have just given birth.
- Physical strength is not the best method of restraint in pigs, but careful, considerate handling and the building of trust is.

Key Points

- Pigs can be dangerous due to their strength and size.
- Pigs have poor eyesight but a very good sense of hearing.
- Physical strength alone cannot restrain a pig.

Self-assessment Questions

1   Why are pigs prone to overheating?

2   How do you build trust with a pig?

3   What is the best way to catch a piglet?

4   How should a group of pigs be moved?

Answers can be found in the back of the book.

References

DEFRA (2003) *Code of Recommendations for the Welfare of Livestock: Pigs*, DEFRA Publications, London.

Edwards, S. (2011) Pigs. In: *Management of Welfare of Farm Animals* (ed J. Webster), John Wiley & Sons Ltd, Chichester, pp. 252–294.

Frantz, L., Meijaard, E., Gongora, J. *et al.* (2016) The evolution of Suidae. *Annual Review of Animal Biosciences*, **4**, 61–85.

Giuffra, E., Kijas, J.M.H., Amarger, V. et al. (2000) The origin of the domestic pig: independent domestication and subsequent introgression. *Genetics*, **154**, 1785–1791.

Lewis, C.R.G. and McGlone, J.J. (2007) Short communication: Moving finishing pigs in different group sizes: Cardiovascular responses, time, and ease of handling. *Livestock Science*, **107**, 86–90. doi: 10.1016/j.livsci.2006.10.011.

Lewis, C.R.G., Hulbert, L.E. and McGlone, J.J. (2008) Short communication: Novelty causes elevated heart rate and immune changes in pigs exposed to handling, alleys, and ramps. *Livestock Science*, **116**, 338–341. doi: 10.1016/j.livsci.2008.02.014.

Rabaste, C., Faucitano, L., Saucier, L. et al. (2007) The effects of handling and group size on welfare of pigs in lairage and their influence on stomach weight, carcass microbial contamination and meat quality. *Canadian Journal of Animal Science*, **87** (1), 3–12. doi: 10.4141/A06-041.

Further Reading

Arbuckle, B.S. (2013) The late adoption of cattle and pig husbandry in Neolithic Central Turkey. *Journal of Archaeological Science*, **40** (4), 1805–1815.

Kittawornrat, A. and Zimmerman, J.J. (2011) Towards a better understanding of pig behaviour and pig welfare. *Animal Health Research Reviews*, **12** (1), 25–32 (http://dx.doi.org/10.1017/S1466252310000174; last accessed 2 June 2017).

12

Handling and Restraint of South American Camelids

Krista M. McLennan[1] and Stella J. Chapman[2]

[1]Chester University, Chester, UK
[2]University Centre Hartpury, Gloucestershire, UK

Members of the camelid family evolved to live in arid and mountainous areas. This chapter focuses on what are known as the New World species of camelid, whose habitat mainly covers the Andes regions of South America.

Four camelids can be found in South America, namely: Guanacos (*Lama guanicoe*), vicunas (*Lama vicugna*), llamas (*Lama guanicoe glama*) and alpacas (*Vicugna pacos*). The two wild forms, the guanaco and the vicuna, diverged from a common ancestor approximately two million years ago, an event unrelated to domestication. Due to hybridization, the exact process of domestication has been controversial, However, recent genetic analysis has suggested that the alpaca is the domesticated form of the vicuna and the llama is the domesticated form of the guanaco (Kadwell *et al.*, 2001). Domestication is thought to have taken place some 6000 years ago (Wheeler, 1995), when a predominant herding economy based on llamas and alpacas was established at Telarmachay (a region of the Peruvian Andes). Archaeological evidence suggests that both llamas and alpacas were part of a sacrificial rite in South American culture and were key to the expansion of the Inca Empire some 500 years ago (Bonacic, 2011).

Physically (apart from size) there is little difference between the llama and alpaca, which is a result of deliberate hybridization between the two species over the past 35 years. Whilst the alpaca and llama still play an important role in their countries of origin, they are also viewed worldwide as: pets, exotic animals, livestock, zoo animals and wild animals.

Alpacas

There are two breeds of alpaca: the Suri alpaca and the Huacaya alpaca. In recent years, for a number of reasons alpacas have become more popular worldwide as a species to either farm or keep as pets. One of the main reasons for farming alpacas is their fine fleece, which is a delicate, lightweight, cashmere-like wool that comes in a range of colours (white, fawn, brown, grey and black). Alpacas have also been bred to protect livestock, particularly sheep.

Llamas

The llama was bred as a pack animal, enabling transport of goods over the mountainous terrain of Peru, Bolivia, Chile and Argentina. They also provide local people with meat, wool and hides for shelters. In common with the alpaca, llamas are also used to protect livestock.

With regards to their welfare, a set of Minimum Standards of Care for Llamas and Alpacas is available (see Further Reading). This sets out the basic requirements that should be considered when keeping these species.

12.1 Behaviour

The domestic camelid still retains much of its wild counterparts' behaviour. Camelids are very sociable, living in small herds and tending to stay together. The camelid is a prey species that is always alert and has very highly developed senses and defence reflexes. This can mean that they can be quite flighty animals and care must be taken to get them used to being handled to avoid stress.

Camelids, similar to other prey species, have a flight zone and a point of balance that can be used when moving a group. They are more likely to flee away from a situation to a safe distance from where they can observe the situation and work out what is the best way to deal with it. If they are unable to flee, such as when they are being restrained or moved into a smaller area, an unhandled or fearful camelid will use its defence system: spitting. Camelids can regurgitate their stomach contents, spitting it towards their advancing attacker. The warning signs include a grumbling and sneezing towards the handler or attacker. If this does not stop the approach, it can bite and kick. Camelids are highly intelligent and intuitive, and a well-handled camelid is calm and easy to handle.

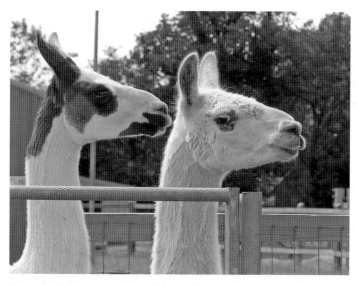

Figure 12.1 Alert ear position of llamas (Source: Courtesy of Brinsbury Campus, Chichester College).

12.1.1 Alpacas and Llama

Alpacas and llamas are herd animals and generally do better if they have other herd mates nearby. In general, llamas are calmer, but for both species ear and tail positions allow both species to express important information about their general emotional state (Figures 12.1, 12.2 and 12.3).

12.2 How to Use Behavioural Traits to Effect When Handling

Due to living as a group, camelids can be herded in a similar way to the other herbivore species (sheep, goats and cattle). The use of dogs and vehicles is not recommended, as this can increase the stress response of camelids more than by using people on foot (Arzamendia *et al.*, 2010). Alpacas are more easily herded than llamas (Bonacic, 2011)

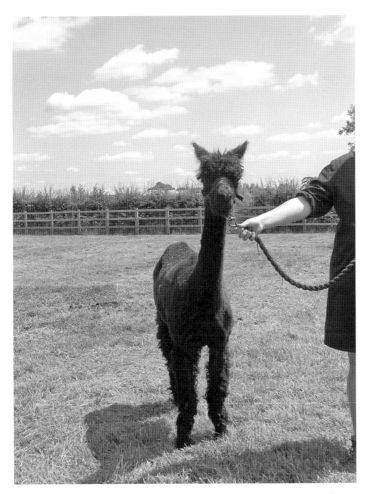

Figure 12.2 Alpaca with ears relaxed and to the side whilst being led in hand and ear positioning changing to being pulled back indicating stress response whilst being more closely handled (Source: Courtesy of Brinsbury Campus, Chichester College).

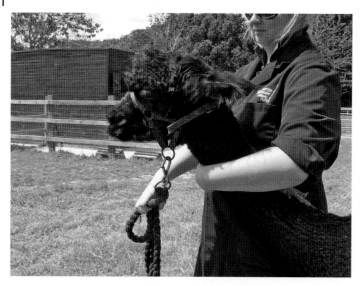

Figure 12.3 Alpaca with ears relaxed and to the side whilst being led in hand and ear positioning changing to being pulled back indicating stress response whilst being more closely handled (Source: Courtesy of Brinsbury Campus, Chichester College).

but both should be worked as a unit rather than as individuals, keeping a group together as much as possible. This will allow the animals to stay calm and, thus, reduces stress. If one animal is needed, herding the group into a handling pen and then separating them into smaller and smaller groups will reduce the stress experienced. When separating off an individual, always keep the group or a small group in close proximity and within sight of the individual being handled. This will keep the animal calm and reduce the likelihood of the animal trying to escape from the area or the restraint.

As with all groups of animals, when moving a group a plan must be in place and all parties involved should know what they are required to do. Any gates that need to be opened, or through which the group needs to go, should be checked before movement begins. When moving a group, use the natural tendency of the camelid to walk away from people. Walk behind them gently with the arms outstretched or with extension wands. Avoid waving arms or wands around, as this can panic them. If there is a group of people, they can help to herd them into a handling pen by using a semicircular motion behind the group with their arms outstretched. Walk slowly towards the group in a calm and confident manner. If you show any hesitation about moving them forward, the alpacas and llamas will become unsure of the situation and more likely to break off. The group should continue to walk away from the handlers and move into the area required (Figure 12.4). When herding the animals continue to use the same principals of the flight zone, point of balance and pressure and release as discussed in Chapter 9.

When handling camelids, it is important to note that in particularly they do not like having their heads touched or handled (Fowler, 2008). It is better to gain control of the neck (Figure 12.5), as this is a very powerful leverage tool and can be easily handled. The camelid does not generally appreciate being fussed over and does better when it is simply supported rather than stroked or touched. Reassure the animal through voice and a calm confident demeanour.

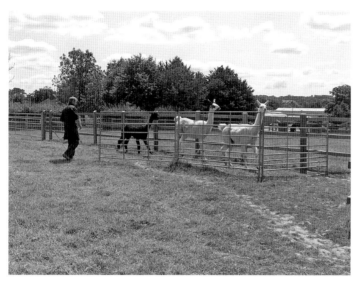

Figure 12.4 Moving camelids into a handling pen in the field (Source: Courtesy of Brinsbury Campus, Chichester College).

12.2.1 Handling Facilities

Before moving any animal or group it is imperative that all facilities have been checked for safety and are fit for purpose. Good handling facilities will include a good sized catch pen and should include a funnel down into a smaller catch pen or chute, where only two or three animals can be contained at one time. These may be permanent or temporary facilities and should be placed in an appropriate area of the field or housing area. The

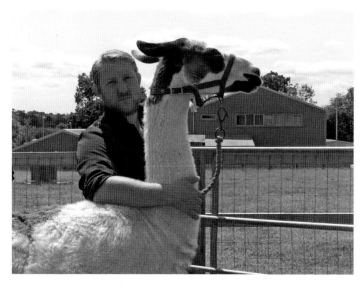

Figure 12.5 Restraint of the neck (Source: Courtesy of Brinsbury Campus, Chichester College).

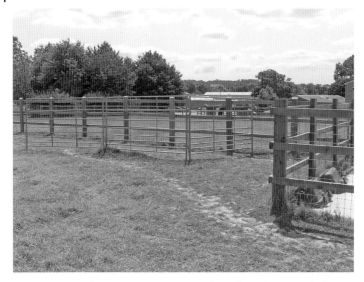

Figure 12.6 Catch pen (Source: Courtesy of Brinsbury Campus, Chichester College).

area should be well lit and well ventilated, ideally with the provision of some form of shelter for adverse weather conditions.

The smaller catch pen (Figure 12.6) allows for the camelids to be contained in an area where they should feel safe and be familiar with. These smaller pens also allow cria to be caught and handled, and are often a good place to start halter training. The pen should enable camelids to see their social group as much as possible.

Chutes or individual corral systems should have shoulder bars to prevent the animal from moving forward and a moveable back bar or board in place to prevent the animal reversing out of the space. A moveable bar or board means that it can be adjusted for each animal depending upon size. If this is in place the animal should not need to be tied up, as they are contained within this area. The animal should only be tied if working alone, making sure that there is enough rope so that if they were to reverse, the camelid would reach the back bar before the rope is pulled. It is imperative that special attention is given to the halter in this case, as there will be no one to correct it should it slip down the nose of the camelid and restrict breathing. It must fit correctly. If the animal is tied, it should be cross-tied with two ropes rather than with a single rope to one side. The sides of the chutes should also be high enough to prevent the animal from trying to escape over the top but not so high that they cannot see out over the top.

12.3 How to Approach and Halter a Camelid

12.3.1 Approaching Adult Camelids

It is easiest to approach a camelid once it has been driven into a smaller area that has been set up for handling. Camelids should be funnelled slowly and calmly into smaller and smaller areas until it is possible to move between the animals without them moving away from the handler. Approach the llama or alpaca preferably from the left side, talking all the time in a calm and gentle voice. Place the left hand at the base of the neck at the front and the right hand on the withers. If the animal moves backwards away from the handler, the right hand can be placed on the hindquarters at the base of the tail.

12.3.2   Approaching Cria

When approaching cria, it is important to keep an eye on the mother and other herd members. As they are a highly protective species and are used as guard animals by some people, approaching a cria can be very dangerous. It is best to approach the mother in the same manner as above, halter her and then approach the cria.

If you are herding a group of camelids that have cria at foot, extra care and attention must be taken to avoid the cria being trampled or squashed by other animals that may panic. If the group is moved slowly and calmly, the movement of the group should go smoothly. In addition, reduce the number of large adults in the smallest group so that the cria are not trampled by them.

12.3.3   How to Put on a Head Collar/Halter

To place a halter on the alpaca or llama, the lead rope of the halter should be placed over the withers so that it comes around the back of the neck. This enables the rope to be used to stop the camelid moving forward if it were to get free of the handler. With the halter in the left hand, the right arm should reach around the back of the neck and grasp the halter such that both hands are now holding the halter. Pull the halter up so that it is slowly and carefully placed over the nose and pulled gently upwards until it reaches the required position and can be fastened (Figures 12.7, 12.8 and 12.9).

Camelids are semi-obligate nasal breathers and do not have a protective piece of bone over their nasal cavity; thus, it is very important that the nose band of a halter is placed

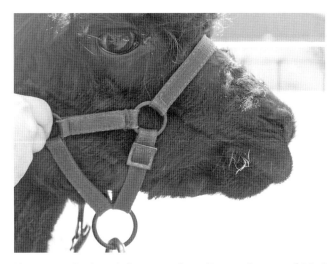

Figure 12.7 Putting a halter on an alpaca (Source: Courtesy of Brinsbury Campus, Chichester College).

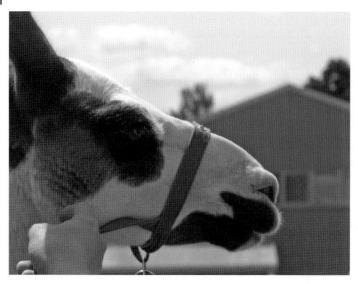

Figure 12.8 Putting a head collar or halter on a llama (Source: Courtesy of Brinsbury Campus, Chichester College).

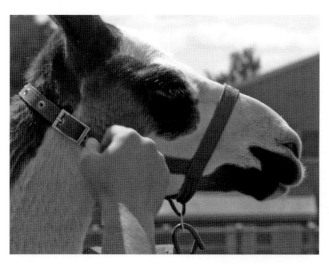

Figure 12.9 Putting a head collar or halter on a llama (Source: Courtesy of Brinsbury Campus, Chichester College).

correctly. If it is too low down on the nose it can prevent the animal from breathing, causing the camelid to suffer.

12.3.4 How to Lead a Camelid

Once a camelid is familiar with a halter, the handler should stand just in front and off to the left side of the animal and increase pressure on the lead rope. As soon as the animal moves forward, release the pressure as a reward. Be calm and use a soft voice, but be

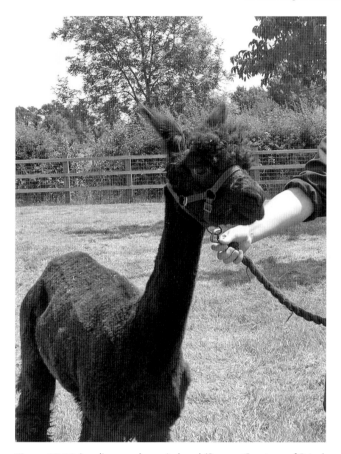

Figure 12.10 Leading an alpaca in hand (Source: Courtesy of Brinsbury Campus, Chichester College).

confident and consistent in your actions, walking forward calmly. Continue the pressure and release until the animal is easily walking beside the handler. The lead rope of the halter should be held so that the right hand is holding the rope a few inches below the chin (Figure 12.10) and the left hand is holding the remainder of the rope.

Never wrap the rope around your hand.

12.4 How to Restrain a Camelid

12.4.1 Methods and Equipment

Before carrying out any restraint for treatment, it is really important to be prepared. This will save time in the long run and can allow you to complete the task much more efficiently, thereby reducing the stress levels in the animal. Camelids do better with less restraint and most camelids can accept general routine treatments without the need for any restraint. They can simply be placed in an area that contains them within a set space, such as a corral or specialized fenced area. If the animal feels safe enough, the handler can simply hold the camelid by a head collar whilst they are within the contained space.

Well-trained and well-handled animals do very well within this containment area rather than being restrained. Animals that fight against restraint need to be handled considerately and excessive pressure should not be applied; instead, time and patience should be given to reassure the animal as much as possible. If further restraint is needed, they should have someone holding them rather than them being in a chute. If the use of a chute is required, it should be designed so that it forms a brace around the shoulder of the camelid and not the head area (Fowler, 2008) as described previously.

Attention should be given to camelids that voluntarily sit down and refuse to move. Kushing (sitting down) is a sign of submission, indignation or displeasure in which they will tuck all their legs tightly under their body (Goplen *et al.*, 2014). However, they can very quickly stand up from this position, so handlers should be aware of this.

If the animal sits down, the task required should be completed as quickly as possible, so they can be left alone and given time to recover. They should not be forced to move. The more they are handled well, the less likely this will happen.

12.4.2 Physical Restraint

A well-trained llama and alpaca can be restrained by simply placing one hand around the front of the neck area and one hand behind the tail and hindquarters (Figure 12.11).

Caution should be taken not to pull or twist the tail but to simply hold it without pressure to begin with. The neck and head area can be pulled into the handler's body for extra support and reassurance to the animal, as well as allowing the handler to get good control of the head and neck. The head is a very powerful area and can cause serious injury if allowed to be used to swing towards the handler. For larger animals such as the llama, if the hindquarters cannot be reached, simple pressure around the withers can steady a well-trained animal. It must be remembered that the necks of camelids are fairly long and if the head is the only point of the animal that is being used for control this can unbalance the

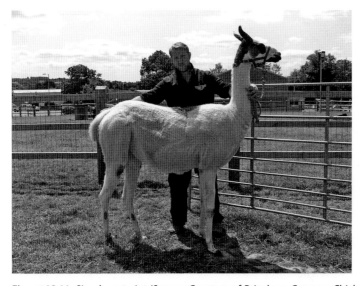

Figure 12.11 Simple restraint (Source: Courtesy of Brinsbury Campus, Chichester College).

animal and cause it some distress. Keeping the head and neck supported, either by hand or by placing a specialized neck wrap around the animal, can help keep the animal calm. If a neck wrap is to be used, instructions on its fitting must be carefully followed and regular checks should be made to ensure that it is fitting correctly without causing any excessive pressure on the neck. Alternatively, the handler can place one hand behind the animal's head with the thumb and forefinger underneath the respective ear, and the other hand under the chin with the thumb and forefingers grasping around the jaw area.

For extra control, a halter can also be placed on the animal, as described above. For larger animals such as llamas, they can be gently pushed against a wall to facilitate the restraint. One hand should be placed on the withers of the animal whilst the other hand controls the head and neck movement. For a secure hold, place the head in the point of the elbow pulling the head and neck towards the body. Both or one of the handlers' legs can be used to gently push the body of the llama into the side of the wall, bracing the back and front legs to prevent movement.

If the above does not steady the animal, one front leg can be placed in a sling secured over the top of the withers of the animal. This will prevent it from moving forward or backwards easily.

For further restraint, the use of a twitch is not advised in camelids, but an ear can be held gently and squeezed at the base. It should never be twisted or pulled, as this can be painful and is highly aversive to the animal. To hold an ear, the handler should stand on the left side of the withers and place the right hand over the neck working the hand up towards the ear (Figure 12.12).

Caution must be taken as the llama may respond by swinging its head towards the left where the handler stands, as they do not like to have their heads handled. This can cause serious injury to both the handler and the animal, and thus this technique should be used with caution and only when absolutely necessary.

If a specially designed chute suitable for use with a llama or alpaca is available, this can be used in cases where holding the animal is not possible for the handler. The camelid can be prevented from moving backwards with a simple bar or rope at the end and a shoulder brace at the front. The use of a cross-tie with two lead ropes attached to the halter can be used to keep the animal in place. If possible the ropes should be held by an assistant rather than tied. This should only be used as a last resort if the shoulder brace does not work.

Smaller animals such as juvenile camelids can be placed in a kushed (sitting) position. Sometimes the animal can be kushed by simply applying pressure to the withers or hindquarters. Alternatively, chukkering (roping) can be used (Fowler, 2008). The handler should stand such that the alpaca is parallel to the legs of the handler. A loose rope is tied around the flank area, cranial to the pelvis. Reaching across the back of the alpaca, the handler should pick up the far hind leg and place the foot in the loop so that it sits ventral to the abdomen. Whilst supporting the alpaca, the handler should place the remaining hind foot into the rope, causing the alpaca to sit down on its back legs. A rope can be placed around the front legs to keep the animal sitting on its sternum.

A juvenile camelid can be restrained in the kush position by a single person straddling (not sitting on) the animal. The handler that is straddling the animal should place one hand on the shoulder to reassure the animal, whilst the other holds the neck just under the chin area to help control the head. If a halter is present, the person straddling the camelid can also hold the collar to help control the head.

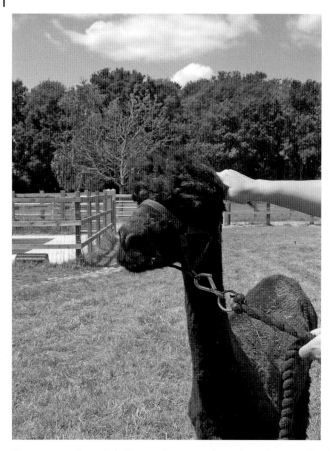

Figure 12.12 Ear twitch (Source: Courtesy of Brinsbury Campus, Chichester College).

If a juvenile needs to be cast so that it is in lateral recumbency, the handler should, with the camelid parallel to the body, reach over the top of the animal and, grasping both limbs on the near side, lift with the knees, allowing the animal to slowly and carefully slide down the body of the handler so that it is placed on its side. The arm holding the foreleg should then be placed over the neck and pressure applied with the elbow. The arm holding the hind limb should be used to apply pressure over the top of the body.

When giving an injection to the animal, do so on the opposite side to where the handler is. This will mean that as the animal moves away from the sensation of the needle, they are moving towards the handler. This will give much better control over the actual injection whilst allowing the animal to have some manoeuvrability.

12.4.3   Training Adult Camelids for Restraint

Training camelids to accept human contact, whether it is simply approaching and holding the animal or leading it by a halter and rope, will take time and patience but will make handling a much better experience for all involved. Camelids are highly intelligent and inquisitive animals and can be easily taught to accept handling and restraint. Having a good understanding of their behaviour, and patience, will go a long way. Camelids respond well to food rewards. They are particularly fond of having a set routine, so daily handling or human contact at the time of feeding will be a great place to start. Increasing the frequency at which they are asked to come in for a small food reward will increase the chances of a good handling and restraint technique being developed. It is possible for camelids to experience veterinary visits, toe trimming and other management practices with very little restraint, if they have been carefully and considerately trained. Providing them with a good experience throughout their daily handling can help to build a good working relationship with the animal, leading to better handling practices all round.

Make sure that any environment used for training is secure and suitable. Young animals should be exposed to and kept with, where possible, older more experienced individuals that can be used to demonstrate to young or nervous animals the benefits of being handled by humans. If time is put into training the animal carefully and with consideration, the camelid should be easy to handle and will require little restraint to carry out everyday tasks.

12.5 Training Cria

When training cria or young to accept and walk on a lead, attach the halter as previously described and start by walking beside them placing a hand on their withers for reassurance. Having a familiar older and more experienced animal with them will encourage them to walk forward and is good practice.

If the cria or young juvenile has not yet been trained to walk on the lead, it can be moved in a similar way to that of a calf or foal, with one hand around the neck/chest area and the other hand wrapped underneath the tail around the hindquarters. They can either be encouraged to walk forward like this or can be carried in this manner if small enough by placing the hand at the back of the animal slightly lower around the hindquarters just above the hocks and lifting the animal off the floor. The cria should be held firmly against the body of the person lifting it so that it feels secure. Alternatively, cria or juvenile camelids can be lifted by placing one hand around the chest with the other hand reaching over the top of the animal and grasping underneath the flank before lifting (Fowler, 2008).

12.6 Special Considerations

- Camelids do not enjoy being touched around the head or being fussed over.
- Stress can be a killer in camelids. Consider when it is time to stop and let the animal recover.
- Training is always best carried out in a safe environment in a calm manner and in small bouts.
- Camelids can kick, bite (large canines) and spit as part of their defence. Placing a towel or piece of cloth over the nose of the camelid is a good way of reducing the chances of

being spat on; however, this can be very stressing, as it can suppress their ability to breathe freely. Standing out of the way or directing the head away from you is a much better alternative.

- Their large powerful necks means that camelids can head fling and cause serious injury to a handler that does not have control of the head and neck area.
- If camelids have cria at foot, during any restraint visual contact should be maintained at all times. This will keep the female much calmer.

Key Points

- Observe the body language of a camelid. If the ears go back and a gurgling sound is heard, this is an indication that they are about to spit.
- Be aware of camelids with cria at foot.
- Make sure that the halter is correctly fitted on a camelid, as it can only breathe through its nose and if the halter is not correctly fitted it can cause the camelid to suffocate.

Self-assessment Questions

1 What is the primary defence reaction of a camelid and what methods can be used to avoid this?

2 What are 'extension wands' used for?

3 Describe the key features of a good handling chute.

4 Outline the importance of a correctly fitting head collar.

5 What is kushing and what are the welfare concerns associated with this?

Answers can be found in the back of the book.

References

Arzamendia, Y., Bonacic, C. and Vilá, B. (2010) Behavioural and physiological consequences of capture for shearing of vicuñas in Argentina. *Applied Animal Behaviour Science*, **125**, 163–170.

Bonacic, C. (2011) South American Camelids. In: *Management and Welfare of Farm Animals* (ed J. Webster), Universities Federation of Animal Welfare (UFAW), Wheathampstead, UK.

Fowler, M. (2008) *Restraint and Handling of Wild and Domestic Animals*, 3rd edn, John Wiley & Sons, Inc, Hoboken, NJ.

Goplen, A.E., Gonzales, S., Ferguson, S. *et al.* (2014) Restraint. In: *Large Animal Medicine for Veterinary Technicians* (eds L. Lien, S. Loly and S. Ferguson), John Wiley & Sons Ltd, Chichester, 29–64.

Kadwell, M., Fernandez, M., Stanley, H.F. *et al.* (2001) Genetic analysis reveals the wild ancestors of the llama and alpaca. *Proceedings of the Royal Biological Society*, **268** (1485), 2575–2584.
Wheeler, J.C. (1995) Evolution and present situation of the South American Camelidae. *Biological Journal of the Linnean Society*, **54** (3), 271–295.

Further Reading

Camelid Community Standards of Care Working Group (2005) Minimum standards of care for llamas and alpacas. https://icinfo.org/sites/camelid-sta.osumc.edu/files/documents/MinimumSOCFINAL.pdf; last accessed 2 June 2017.
Christman, J. (2010) Physical methods of capture, handling and restraint of mammals. In: *Wild Mammals in Captivity. Principles and Techniques of Zoo Management* (eds D.G. Kleiman, K.V. Thompson and C. Kirk Baer), 2nd edn, The University of Chicago Press, Chicago, IL, pp. 39–48.
The British Alpaca Society (ND) https://www.bas-uk.com/; last accessed 2 June 2017.

13

Handling and Restraint of Poultry and Aviary Birds

William S.M. Justice[1] and Stella J. Chapman[2]

[1]*Marwell Wildlife, Winchester, UK*
[2]*University Centre Hartpury, Gloucestershire, UK*

The chicken (*Gallus domesticus*) was first domesticated about 8000 years ago from a wild form known as the red junglefowl (*Gallus gallus*), which still runs wild in most of Southeast Asia and was most likely hybridized with the grey junglefowl (*Gallus sonneratii*). The chicken is the most widespread domesticated animal found around the world; however, the timings and locations of their domestication are controversial. Some authors suggest that the earliest archaeological evidence is from China around 5400 BC. However, recent genetic evidence suggests that further analysis, including mDNA studies, are required in order to fully reveal the origin and history of the domestic chicken (Eda *et al.*, 2016).

It is important to mention that whilst a timeline for the domestication of chickens is provided, people keep indoor and aviary birds for many reasons and recently the term non-traditional companion animals (NTCA) has started to be used, rather than the term 'exotics' to describe their position as a 'pet' animal rather than as a domesticated animal. The British Veterinary Association (BVA) has recently developed a policy statement in association with the British Small Animal Veterinary Association (BSAVA), British Veterinary Zoological Society (BVZS) and the Fish Veterinary Society (FVS). Under this policy, NTCAs are considered as those animals that are not traditionally kept as pets in the United Kingdom and, as such, their 'five welfare needs' are so specialized that they could rarely or never be met in a domestic environment (BVA, 2015).

Each year, the Pet Food Manufacturers Association (PFMA) conducts a survey in the United Kingdom that looks at pet ownership trends. In 2015, it was estimated that 1% of households in the United Kingdom owned a total of 0.7 million domestic fowl (i.e. chickens) and 0.5 million indoor birds (PFMA, 2015).

For the purpose of this chapter, any reference to poultry will refer to backyard poultry only, that is those kept in small groups by private owners. Poultry and aviary birds are often kept in a domestic setting and, consequently, may be used to the presence of people on a daily routine. It should not be assumed, however, that these birds are domesticated in the same sense that a pet cat or dog is – true domestication of a species is a lengthy process that can take many generations to achieve. There is a great diversity in the species of birds kept in aviaries, ranging from small passerines, such as canaries, to

Safe Handling and Restraint of Animals: A Comprehensive Guide, First Edition. Stella J. Chapman.
© 2018 John Wiley & Sons Ltd. Published 2018 by John Wiley & Sons Ltd.

psittacines like budgerigars. Handling principles for the different species have much in common, though there are several differences, depending on size and species.

13.1   Behavioural Considerations

In most cases, poultry and aviary birds are prey species. In nature, these birds would never be 'handled' by another species unless caught by a predator and, therefore, it should be assumed that handling is generally a stressful experience for birds, particularly if they are not used to people. This should still be a consideration even when birds are handled routinely and appropriate steps should be taken to reduce the likelihood of causing unnecessary stress to an individual.

13.1.1   Flight Distance

For most species a flight distance exists. This is the minimum distance a potential threat can be from the bird before it alters its behaviour to increase that distance, generally by flying or running away. This distance can be reduced through habituating the bird to the presence of people, though this should be done gradually in a step-wise fashion to avoid any negative experience.

13.1.2   Environment

Once in the hand, most birds will attempt to escape given the smallest of opportunities. In many cases birds will attempt to fly away, often towards the most obvious exit. For this reason it is very important to consider the surroundings prior to handling birds. Birds should be handled in an enclosed area, making sure doors and windows are shut and that there are no high places, for example the tops of cupboards, where they can get out of reach of handlers. Closed windows still present a significant risk, as birds will fly into them in an effort to escape, sometimes sustaining injury in the process. To avoid this, it is useful to pull blinds, draw curtains or use another method to block the light from windows. Take care if other people or animals are in the vicinity to avoid inadvertent injury to the bird if it escapes.

13.2   Anatomical Considerations

Birds have a unique anatomy adapted to flight. It is important to be aware of several features that can have a bearing on handling techniques.

Skeleton
The skeleton has several adaptions.

- The cervical vertebrae are generally flexible, allowing a good range of motion for feeding.
- In general, the thoracic vertebrae are fused, as are the lumbar vertebrae and pelvis forming the sacrum.

- The caudal vertebral bones form the pygostyle, which supports the tail feathers.
- The skeleton takes a heavy impact when birds land and the fused vertebrae provide extra support to counteract this.

Wings
- Wings are similar to the forelimb of mammals, consisting of shoulder, elbow and carpal joints, with three digits forming the wing tip.
- Wings should normally fold up against the body so that the elbow and wing tip point towards the back of the bird.

Respiratory System
- The respiratory system is also unique and allows gas exchange to occur very efficiently, providing birds with the oxygen needed to sustain the high metabolic rate needed for flight.
- Most birds breathe through their nares, the openings into the nasal passages, which sit on either side of the upper portion of the beak.
- Open mouth breathing is uncommon and can often be a sign of stress or disease. If this is seen, handling should be avoided unless absolutely essential.
- The trachea is made up of complete rings of cartilage, unlike in mammals where they are incomplete. This provides the trachea with some rigidity, which means that the risk of accidently obstructing the airway is less likely compared with mammals.
- The lungs of birds are rigid structures that do not inflate and collapse with each breath. Instead, air sacs both in front of and behind the lungs, inflate and collapse as the bird breathes, thus driving air through the lung structure. These air sacs are situated around the body organs making them relatively easy to compress by external forces. Handlers should be aware that if they grip too hard around the main body of a bird, this will restrict air flow through the lungs and compromise the bird's ability to breathe.

Beak
- The beak is made up of supporting bones covered with a layer of keratin.
- This light weight structure replaces the heavy jaw bone and dentition of mammals, though at the expense of certain actions, for example chewing, which is functionally replaced by a muscular stomach that helps grind up food material.
- Consequently, birds do not have teeth, but in some cases (e.g. parrots) can still use their beak very effectively to inflict injury on a handler when defending themselves.

Gastrointestinal Tract (GIT)
- The GIT terminates at the cloaca, which is also the terminal point for the urinary and genital tracts.
- All products from these tracts exit the bird via a single opening, known as the vent.
- Handlers should be aware of its position and that birds void urates and faeces when handled.

Feathers
- All birds have feathers, which may be involved in a variety of different functions including flight, thermoregulation, reproductive displays and waterproofing/buoyancy.

- Birds spend a significant proportion of their behavioural repertoire looking after their feathers, a process known as preening, often coating them with an oily secretion from their preen gland, which is located at the base of their tail (not present in all species).
- This gives some indication as to the importance of good feather condition to the welfare of birds.
- It should be noted that feathers can easily be damaged during handling, with disruption ranging from separation of the individual barbs located on the feather shaft to loss of several feathers. Given the critical importance of feathers to certain functions, this can potentially have a significant impact on the welfare of the bird.
- All birds moult out old feathers and replace them with new ones, usually sequentially to mitigate any impacts on function whilst this occurs. As new feathers grow they appear as short, highly vascularized shafts known as blood feathers. Great care should be taken not to damage these feather shafts during handling as they can bleed profusely. As the feather matures, the blood supply is withdrawn, so there is no risk of bleeding from mature feathers if the shaft is broken. However, handlers should bear in mind that if mature feathers are broken off, the remaining portion of the feather shaft can have a particularly sharp end, which may be a hazard for both the bird and handler.

13.3 How to Restrain Birds

13.3.1 Preparation Prior to Handling

As previously discussed, it should be assumed that handling any bird may involve some degree of stress for that individual. Steps should be taken to reduce the impact on welfare as much as possible. To this end:

- Any handling event should be planned in advance with a clear goal of what the handler is trying to achieve, for example moving an individual to another enclosure.
- The time the bird is kept in hand should be kept to the minimum amount needed to complete the task.
- Any equipment needed should be made ready and be easily accessible to the handler.
- Stress can be minimized by using a quiet, dark location for handling.
- The handling area should be away from any potential predators.
- Any doors and windows should be shut and blinds or curtains drawn to prevent birds flying at a closed window in the event they escape from the handlers' grip.
- Locations should also be chosen that allow easy recapture, should this be necessary.

13.3.2 Visual Assessment of Birds

Birds should be assessed visually prior to handling. Some may already show high levels of stress as a result of a change in routine, for example being corralled into a small area, or the presence of multiple people or capture equipment involved in the procedure. These birds will often be flying back and forth between perching areas in a high state of alert and may be breathing open mouthed when perched. In these cases it is usually best to allow the bird to settle down before handling is attempted. This may mean a delay of 30–60 minutes (or longer) to allow the bird to get used to the change in circumstances.

The acclimatization can be expedited by making the area darker and quiet. This may mean turning off lights in a room or placing a towel over three sides of the cage to remove any perceived threats and make the bird feel safer.

Birds that are unwell are often perched predominantly in one place and tend not to use the space available to them. Their feathers are often 'fluffed up' as part of the thermoregulatory response to illness and they may also be breathing open mouthed. In this case, no attempt should be made to handle the bird unless absolutely necessary, as birds with respiratory compromise can die as a result. Veterinary advice should be sought immediately.

13.4 Handling Techniques for Common Cage and Aviary Species

13.4.1 General Points Regarding the Handling of Poultry

The majority of backyard poultry tends to include chickens, turkeys, ducks and geese. They are often referred to as 'domestic fowl', although the degree of domestication varies by species and, as previously discussed, care should be taken not to assume they are habituated to people. Handlers should be aware of species differences, including 'danger points' such as beak or claw that may cause injury:

- Chickens and turkeys have short narrow beaks adapted to their granivorous diet. If they are used to being handled, they rarely use their beaks to defend themselves. Likewise, they can have sharp claws on their feet, which may cause inadvertent injury to the handler.
- Cockerels are worth a special mention as they have long, sharp spurs on the inside of their leg, just above the foot. These are used for fighting other cockerels in territory disputes, but particularly aggressive cockerels will also attack people if they feel threatened, or if hens are nearby.
- Ducks and geese have broad bills adapted for grazing and filtering food from the water. Larger waterfowl, such as geese, can inflict a painful bite but are unlikely to cause serious damage. Each webbed foot has short claws present; however, these are unlikely to cause a problem for the handler, provided they are wearing suitable clothing.

13.4.2 Handling and Restraint of Chickens

In general:

1) Chickens should be approached from behind and grasped around the shoulders and main part of the wings to keep them against the body (Figures 13.1 to 13.4).
2) The handlers' thumbs should be on top, pointing towards the base of the neck, and remaining fingers underneath (Figure 13.5) gently clasping the legs between the fourth and fifth fingers (though this may vary depending on the size of the chicken).
3) If the wings escape the handlers' grasp, this is normally because their hands are too far back. Flapping wings can be brought under control again by bringing a hand in from in front of the wing and folding it up against the body wall again. The head does not normally need to be restrained (Figure 13.6).

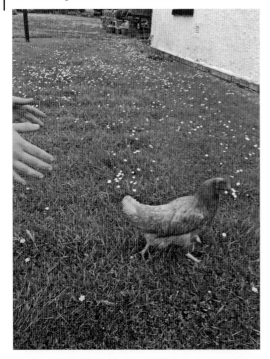

Figure 13.1 Approaching a chicken (Source: Courtesy of Krista McLennan, 2016).

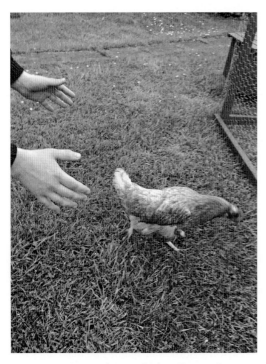

Figure 13.2 Approaching a chicken (Source: Courtesy of Krista McLennan, 2016).

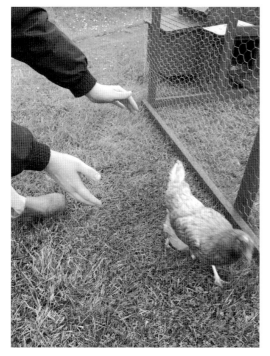

Figure 13.3 Approaching a chicken (Source: Courtesy of Krista McLennan, 2016).

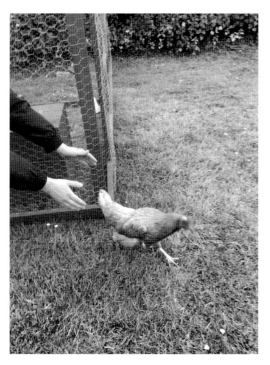

Figure 13.4 Approaching a chicken (Source: Courtesy of Krista McLennan, 2016).

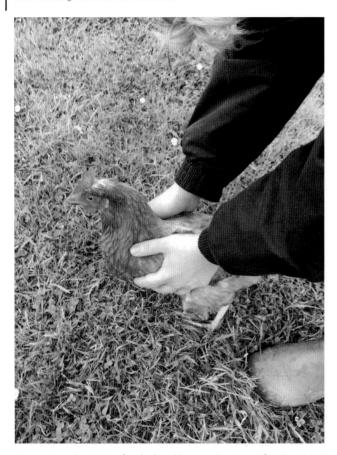

Figure 13.5 Restraint of a chicken (Source: Courtesy of Krista McLennan, 2016).

4) If a wing needs to be examined, it may be easier to hold the chicken against the handler's body. To examine the right wing (Figure 13.7) the chicken is turned to face left and tucked into the crook of the handler's left arm, restrained by the left hand, which comes around the front of the chicken and holds the main body and legs. The right hand is then free to gently extend the right wing out for examination. The left wing can be examined in a similar fashion by facing the chicken to the right and using the right arm to restrain it against the body.

13.4.3   Handling and Restraint of Other Poultry

In general:

- Ducks can be restrained using the same method as chickens.
- Larger birds, such as geese, should always be held against the handler's body, with one arm over the top of the bird's back, holding both wings in place against the bird's body.
- In long necked species this leaves the other hand free to gently control the head and neck by loosely grasping the neck about two-thirds of the way up. This is primarily to prevent pecks to the handler's face and body.

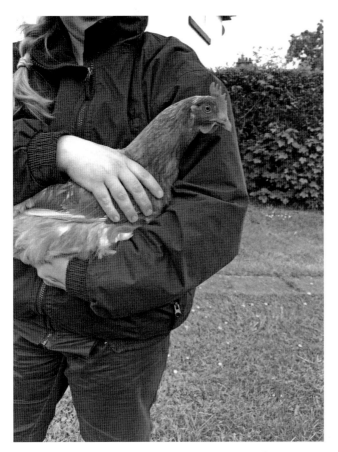

Figure 13.6 Restraint of a chicken (Source: Courtesy of Krista McLennan, 2016).

- Alternatively, the head and neck can be placed under one arm such that the bird is facing in the opposite direction to the handler. The same arm is used to hold the front half of the bird against the handler's body and the other arm is used to restrain the legs (Figure 13.8).

13.4.4 Handling and Restraint of Pigeons and Doves

Pigeons may be kept for a variety of reasons. Racing pigeons are often used to being handled routinely by people and, consequently, may be less stressed by handling. In other situations, such as the breeding of rare species for conservation purposes, excessive human contact may be counterproductive to conservation goals. Consequently, a 'hands-off' approach to management may be taken and these birds are likely to find any kind of handling very stressful. Although pigeons have a short pointed beak and small claws, they generally do not present a high risk to handlers. In general:

- Pigeons should be handled with two hands to minimize the risk of escaping the handler or damaging themselves by attempting to escape (Figures 13.9 and 13.10).

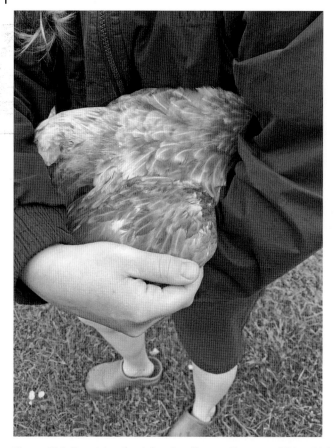

Figure 13.7 Examining the right wing (Source: Courtesy of Krista McLennan, 2016).

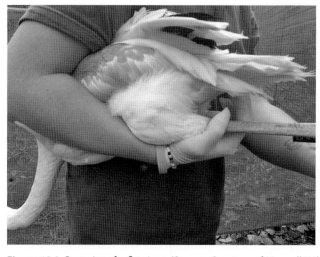

Figure 13.8 Restraint of a flamingo (Source: Courtesy of Marwell Wildlife, 2016).

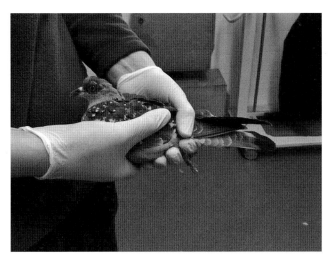

Figure 13.9 Two different approaches to restraining a pigeon (Source: Courtesy of Marwell Wildlife, 2016).

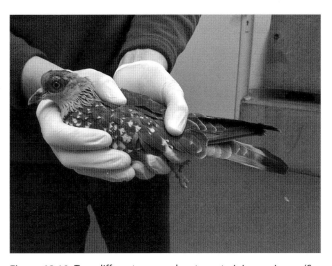

Figure 13.10 Two different approaches to restraining a pigeon (Source: Courtesy of Marwell Wildlife, 2016).

- They are generally best approached from the back and initially held around the wings to keep them against the body.
- The bird may be turned to the left and the pectoral muscles and carpal joints are cupped in the left hand, whilst the thumb of the right hand is placed over the back of the bird holding both wing tips against the body. The second and third fingers of the right hand can then be used to grip the tail feathers and the fourth and fifth fingers can gently restrain the legs. In this way, the flight and tail feathers are relatively protected, reducing the risk of damage during handling. The grip can be reversed depending on what the handler feels most comfortable with.

- To examine the wings, the right hand grip remains the same but the bird is turned towards the handler and held against the body. This frees up the left hand to gently extend the bird's right wing. It is usually best to change hands and reverse the grip in order to examine the left wing.

13.4.5   Handling and Restraint of Small Passerines

Small passerines belong to the order of Passeriformes and consist of many of the familiar garden bird species/songbirds. The canary is an example of one of the more common species kept in captivity. Small passerines are easily stressed by handling. Their small size and high metabolic rate make them very susceptible to physiological stress and it should be noted that small birds can die as a result of handling, even when the handler has taken great care to minimize stress. Small passerines are generally not considered to pose a high risk to the handler and the following points should be noted:

- As with other birds, it is best to approach from behind.
- A single hand can be used to hold the bird over the back with the wings gently held next to the body (Figures 13.11 and 13.12).
- Great care must be taken not to restrict respiratory movement.
- The head can be gently restrained between the first and second fingers, with the thumb and/or fourth and fifth fingers brought around the front of the body in what is commonly referred to as a 'ringers grip' (Whitworth *et al.*, 2007). Both wings can be gently examined using the other hand.

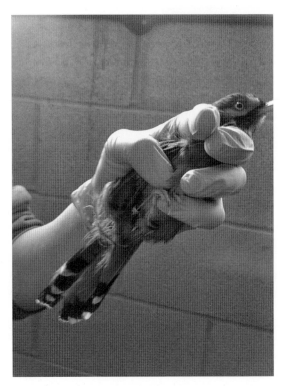

Figure 13.11 Restraint of small passerines (Source: Courtesy of Marwell Wildlife, 2016).

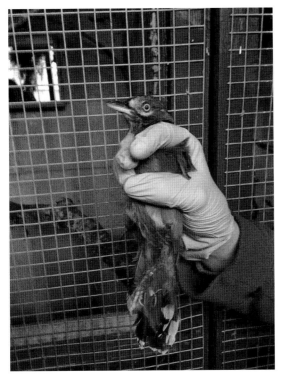

Figure 13.12 Restraint of small passerines (Source: Courtesy of Marwell Wildlife, 2016).

- Alternatively, a small lightweight flannel can be used to restrain the wings against the body of the bird. This allows the bird's head to be covered, which may be helpful in reducing stress. However, if the purpose of handling is examination, the presence of the flannel may become a hindrance as visualizing the whole bird is difficult.
- Larger passerines can be restrained in a similar fashion to medium sized psittacines, as described in the next section.

13.4.6 Handling and Restraint of Psittacines

Many different parrot species are commonly kept in captivity. Pet birds may be well habituated to being handled by people and are very compliant when it comes to handling, often comfortably sitting on an arm or shoulder and making no attempt to fly away. Parrots kept in larger aviaries may not be used to being handled and these, particularly in large species, can present some difficulties when it comes to handling.

Parrots generally have strong beaks, with the upper beak tapering to a sharp point. The upper beak also forms a joint with the bones of the skull, giving some degree of movement. This allows parrots a wide gape and the ability to manipulate their food – an adaptation to eating fruit in the wild. Large species, such as macaws, have very strong beaks adapted for opening nuts. These birds can inflict serious injury on handlers and should only be handled by the experienced.

Many species of parrot commonly kept in captivity can be very amenable to handling. In these cases they may be trained to step up onto a hand or arm when presented. This still needs to be carried out in a safe and secure environment should the bird attempt to fly. However, it has the advantage of greatly reducing the stress involved in handling.

If the individual is not used to handling or is not compliant, for example for behavioural or health reasons, it may be gently restrained.

- In all cases a towel can be very useful for aiding handling and reducing stress.
- Small psittacines do not post a high risk to handlers and can be restrained in much the same way as small passerines using a 'ringers grip' (see previously).
- Larger psittacines are capable of inflicting injury on a handler, so the head needs to be controlled.
- In medium sized birds, the bird is usually approached from behind. The head is gently grasped on either side, where the lower beak meets the skull, using the thumb and first or second finger of the handler's dominant hand. Placement of finger and thumb is important to allow control over the bird's head and avoid bite injury without causing

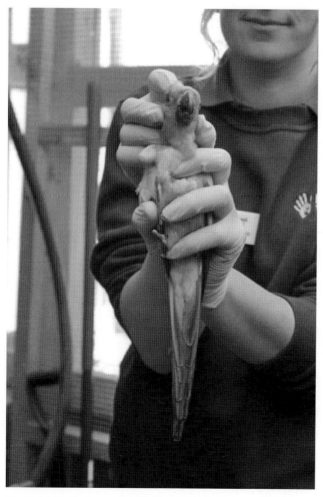

Figure 13.13 Restraint of medium sized psittacine (Source: Courtesy of Marwell Wildlife, 2016).

excessive discomfort. The other hand is used to grip around the back of the bird and support the legs, keeping the wings gently folded in against the body (Figure 13.13)

- Try to avoid putting your hand in front of the bird, as they are more likely to grasp hold of it with their claws and bite should you lose control of the head.
- The legs can also be supported or gently restrained between the third, fourth and fifth fingers depending on the size of the bird.
- A slight variation on this grip involves turning the lower hand to 'cup' the bird from underneath, supporting the back against the handlers' body, allowing the fingers to grip the legs. In this case, the second and fourth fingers are placed around the outside of the legs with the third finger in between to keep them separate. This position has the advantage of ensuring that the legs are not traumatized during handling but the disadvantage is that, in larger birds, there is less control over the wings. To assist with this, a suitably sized towel can be used to keep the wings in place.
- Towels (Figure 13.14) may also be useful for loosely covering the head to help reduce stress. They also provide some protection against bite injury to the handler. Large psittacines, such as macaws, can be handled using this technique, although often two towels are used together to help protect the handler and the head may need to be restrained with the first and second finger opposing the thumb.

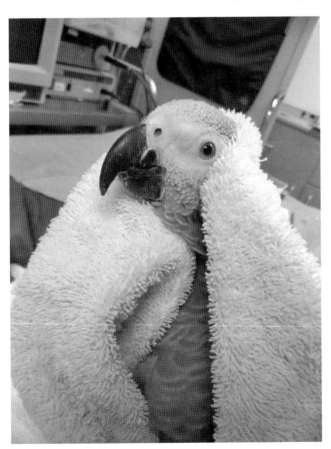

Figure 13.14 Towel restraint of a medium sized psittacine (Source: Courtesy of Wendy Bament).

- Positive reinforcement training has also been used with psittacines to allow them to be handled with minimal stress to the bird.

Key Points

- It should be assumed that handling is a stressful process for most birds. Keep handling to as short a time as necessary and choose a dark, quiet environment where possible to help reduce stress.
- Consider the behavioural and anatomical variations unique to birds and be aware of them when handling.
- Check the environment for potential hazards or escape points carefully before attempting to handle.
- Observe individuals carefully prior to handling to ensure they are not already stressed or unwell.
- Choose a handling technique appropriate to the size and species of bird you are dealing with.

Self-assessment Questions

1 Why is it important to draw curtains or pull blinds in the room before handling birds?

2 Why is it important to not hold birds too tightly around the body?

3 Why should birds be visually assessed prior to handling?

4 Describe a grip commonly used to restrain passerines.

Answers can be found in the back of the book.

References

BVA (2015) Policy statement on non-traditional companion animals. https://www.bva.co.uk/uploadedFiles/Content/News,_campaigns_and_policies/Policies/Companion_animals/non-traditional-companion-animal-policy-position.pdf; last accessed 2 June 2017.

Eda, M., Lu, P., Kikuchi, H. *et al.* (2016) Re-evaluation of early Holocene chicken domestication in northern China. *Journal of Archaeological Science*, **67**, 25–31.

PFMA (2015) Pet Population Statistics 2014–15. Pet Food Manufacturers Association, London (http://www.pfma.org.uk/pet-population-2015; last accessed 2 June 2017).

Whitworth, D., Newman, S., Mundkur, T. and Harris, P. (2007) Bird handling and ringing techniques. In: *Wild Birds and Avian Influenza: An Introduction to Applied Field Research and Disease Sampling Techniques*, Food and Agriculture Organization of the United Nations (FAO), Rome, pp. 51–72.

Further Reading

Chitty, J. and Lierz, M. (2008) *BSAVA Manual of Raptors, Pigeons and Passerine Birds.* British Small Animal Veterinary Association, Gloucester, UK.

Fowler, M.E. (2008) *Restraint and Handling of Wild and Domestic Animals*, 3rd edn, John Wiley & Sons, Inc, Hoboken, NJ.

Fowler, M.E. and Miller, R.E. (2003) *Zoo and Wild Animal Medicine*, 5th edn, Saunders Elsevier.

Girling, S.J. (2013) *Veterinary Nursing of Exotic Pets*, 2nd edn, John Wiley & Sons Ltd, Chichester.

Heard, D.J. (1997) Avian respiratory anatomy and physiology. *Seminars in Avian and Exotic Pet Medicine*, **6** (4), 172–179.

Noble, S., Proctor and Lynch, P.J. (1993) *Manual of Ornithology: Avian Structure and Function*. Yale University Press, New Haven, CT.

Samour, J. (2007) *Avian Medicine*, 2nd edn, Mosby, Maryland Heights, MO.

Withers, P.C. (1992) *Comparative Animal Physiology*, Brooks/Cole–Thomson Learning.

14

Handling and Restraint of Reptiles

William S.M. Justice[1] and Stella J. Chapman[2]

[1]*Marwell Wildlife, Winchester, UK*
[2]*University Centre Hartpury, Gloucestershire, UK*

The term non-traditional companion animals (NTCA) has started to be used, rather than the term 'exotics', to describe their position as a companion animal rather than as a domesticated animal. The British Veterinary Association (BVA) has recently developed a policy statement in association with the British Small Animal Veterinary Association (BSAVA), British Veterinary Zoological Society (BVZS) and the Fish Veterinary Society (FVS). Under this policy NTCAs are considered as those animals, that are not traditionally kept as pets in the United Kingdom and as such their 'five welfare needs' are so specialized that they could rarely or never be met in a domestic environment (BVA, 2015)

Each year, the Pet Food Manufacturers Association (PFMA) conducts a survey in the United Kingdom that looks at pet ownership trends. In 2015, it was estimated that 1% of households in the United Kingdom owned a total of 0.3 million lizards, 0.3 million snakes and 0.2 million tortoises and turtles (PFMA, 2015).

Reptiles are a diverse group. There are four taxonomic groups: squamata (lizards and snakes), chelonia (tortoises and turtles), crocodilia (crocodiles, alligators and gharials) and sphenodontia (only one species, the tuatara). Many are kept as pets by private owners although, like many of the non-traditional companion animals, reptiles are generally not considered domesticated. As most reptiles would not be picked up by another animal in the wild unless predated, it seems reasonable to assume that handling may induce a stress response in most cases. For many of the commonly kept species, regular handling from a young age may help reduce this response but handlers should always be aware of the negative impact they may be having and handle animals with the respect and care they deserve.

There are many techniques for handling reptiles and the more commonly used ones are outlined below. Each groups' characteristic morphology and behaviour determines the method employed for handling.

Legislation

It is worth noting that most tortoises and some other reptiles are listed on Appendix 1 of the Convention on the International Trade in Endangered Species (CITES). This means that they need an appropriate certificate in order to be sold or moved across

Safe Handling and Restraint of Animals: A Comprehensive Guide, First Edition. Stella J. Chapman.
© 2018 John Wiley & Sons Ltd. Published 2018 by John Wiley & Sons Ltd.

international borders. Additionally, in the United Kingdom, some reptiles, for example venomous snakes and crocodilians, need a license to be kept privately under the Dangerous Wild Animals Act (1976).

14.1   Behaviour and Special Considerations

The entire repertoire of reptile behaviours is not fully understood. However, this area of study is growing and the most recent views suggest that behaviours are as complex in reptiles as any other taxonomic group, when given the opportunity to express them. Handlers should at least be aware of the main aggressive and defensive behaviours that reptiles show.

14.1.1   Lizards

Perhaps the most extreme of these behaviours is the ability of some lizards to drop their tail in response to a threat, a process known as **tail autotomy**. These species may have fracture planes present in their tail vertebrae that allow tail separation to occur very rapidly. The tail often continues to twitch for a short time after autotomy has occurred, distracting a potential predator and allowing the lizard time to escape. Great care should be taken when handling lizards to avoid this. The tail will eventually regrow; however, the appearance of the scales (both in size and colour) is usually different to the original. Consequently, lizards should never be handled by the tail.

Other defensive behaviours include inflating the lungs to give themselves the appearance of being larger than they actually are. Tail flicking or whipping is a defensive behaviour used to deter potential predators. In large lizards, tail whipping can inflict a painful injury on the handler; therefore it is usually advisable to use a suitable restraint that prevents this occurring (see below). Head bobbing, in iguanas, is normally a sign of territorial aggression and should be taken as an indicator that an individual feels threatened by your presence.

Occasionally, lizards will bite to defend themselves, though the potential to inflict injury depends on the species. Some lizards, for example Gila monsters, are venomous; therefore, bites from these species can be very serious. These species require special handling techniques (Figure 14.1), an appropriate antivenin (if available) and help nearby in case of a bite injury.

14.1.2   Snakes

Snakes are capable of inflicting bite injuries on handlers but will often give some warning by coiling into a strike position first. However, generally they try to escape any potential threats by moving away and finding a suitable hiding place.

They will occasionally pass foul smelling urates and faeces when they are feeling threatened, presumably to deter potential predators. They may also regurgitate any recently ingested food and, for this reason, snakes should not be handled within 24 hours of feeding.

It is also important to note whether a snake is going into 'shed'. In most species, the scales become dull and the spectacle covering the eye may look opaque. Snakes may be

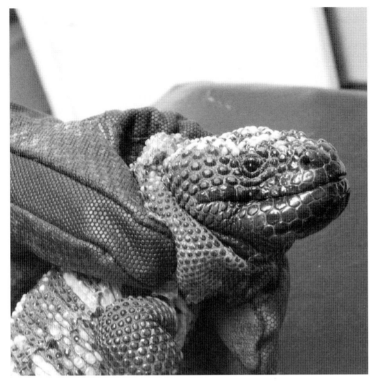

Figure 14.1 Handling a Gila monster with bite proof gloves (Source: Courtesy of Marwell Zoo, 2016).

more defensive during this time, possibly due to reduced vision. Therefore, it is best to avoid handling them until the shed is completed.

14.1.3 Chelonians

Tortoises will generally retreat into their shell when threatened, using their heavily scaled, muscular forelegs to protect their head. As this can impede any kind of close inspection or examination, tortoises should be handled in a way to minimize the chances of this occurring (see below). In some cases, as they pull their head back into their shell, tortoises will exhale rapidly, producing a loud hiss to deter predators. Similar to snakes, tortoises will often pass faeces and urates if they feel threatened.

14.2 Restraint and Handling of Snakes

14.2.1 Anatomical Considerations

Snakes have several unique anatomical adaptations.

- They have strong muscular bodies, which allows locomotion without limbs. Four different types of locomotion exist, namely: lateral undulation, rectilinear locomotion, concertina locomotion and sidewinding. It can be helpful to know which type of locomotion is employed by a species, as handlers can more easily predict the animal's movements.

- The snake skeleton is primarily composed of the skull, spinal column and associated ribs. The ribs provide support and protection for soft tissues along virtually the entire length of the animal. Despite the musculature overlying the ribs, handlers should be aware that individual ribs can be fractured through inappropriate handling techniques, particularly in smaller species. The atlanto-occipital joint (the joint between the skull and vertebral column) is also relatively weak in smaller species and care should be taken, particularly when restraining the head.
- The musculoskeletal anatomy of snakes makes them very flexible and able to turn around in very small spaces. Their muscular strength and smooth scales can make them a challenge to restrain, though this can be overcome using the techniques described in the next section.
- Constrictors have two rows of teeth on their upper jaw and a single row on the lower jaw, all with needle-like backward pointing teeth. This adaptation makes it very difficult for prey to escape once captured. Handlers should be aware of this in case they themselves are accidently bitten, as pulling away can cause trauma to both the snake and the handler.

14.2.2 Handling Snakes

The temperament of snakes can vary by species and individual animal. How amenable they are to handling can often depend on how regularly handling takes place. If a snake is unfamiliar to you, it is always best to use a degree of caution. Always make sure you know what species you are handling and if it is venomous or non-venomous.

14.2.2.1 Non-venomous Snakes

Non-venomous snakes generally use constriction to kill their prey. Small constrictors rarely pose a serious threat to handlers, although they can still deliver a nasty bite if provoked. Large constrictors can be very dangerous due to their strength. A good rule of thumb is to have one person present for every metre of the snake being handled (Figure 14.2).

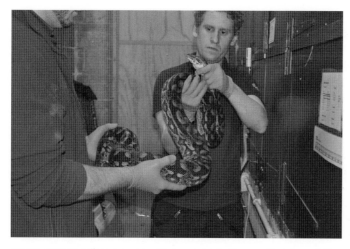

Figure 14.2 Handling a snake with two people (Source: Courtesy of Marwell Wildlife, 2016).

Constrictors should always be handled respectfully and never placed across the shoulders or around the neck.

Snakes should be observed carefully for any signs of aggressive or other abnormal behaviours before handling. They should also be checked to make sure they are not going into shed or that they have not eaten within the last 48 hours.

Remove any items from the snake's immediate environment that may make it difficult to pick them up. It is often useful to let the snake know you are there prior to picking it up. With unfamiliar animals it is usually best to do this by gently touching them with a snake hook or other suitable object that allows you to keep out of striking distance. Always approach them from behind the head to avoid them feeling threatened. If there is little or no reaction to touching with a snake hook, it may be safe to pick up.

- Start by gently grasping the snake's body near the head and lift, then pick up the rest of the snake's body with the other hand/arm.
- Arboreal species like pythons would normally anchor their body by wrapping around a tree branch in the wild. Consequently, when handling they will feel more secure if you let them wrap their tail around your arm (Figure 14.3).
- Use your other hand to keep control of the head, but if the snake is relaxed and wants to explore the environment do not restrict its movement completely, as it is likely to become agitated.
- Allow the snake to move a little through your hand and then reposition it to bring the head back under control. Hold it close to your body, as it will appreciate the warmth and security.
- Where possible, hold the snake over a table, so that there is not a large distance should it fall.
- When placing back into an enclosure or vivarium, place it gently on the floor to allow it to find its own way around or into any furniture items.

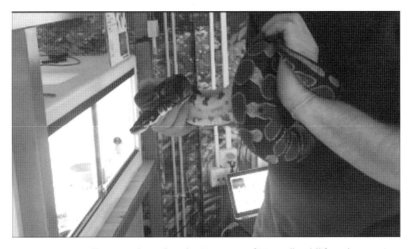

Figure 14.3 Handling an arboreal snake (Courtesy of Marwell Wildlife to be consistent, 2016).

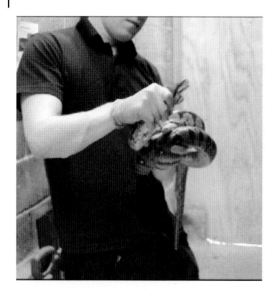

Figure 14.4 Handling an aggressive snake (Source: Courtesy of Marwell Wildlife, 2016).

14.2.2.2 Venomous Snakes

Only experienced people should handle aggressive or venomous species (Figure 14.4).

Antivenin, appropriate for the species being handled, along with an emergency bite protocol should always be available when handling venomous species. Due to potential for serious harm or death from snake bites, these species should only be handled where help is available.

Snake hooks (Figure 14.5) can be used to move snakes whilst keeping the handler beyond striking distance. Hooks should be used in conjunction with the snake's natural movement to help guide them in a specific direction, or gently lift the snake short distances.

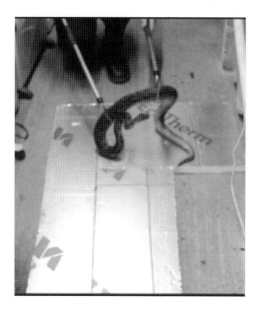

Figure 14.5 Use of snake hooks (Source: Courtesy of Marwell Wildlife, 2016).

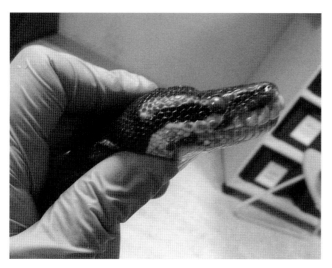

Figure 14.6 Restraint of the head (Source: Courtesy of Marwell Wildlife, 2016).

Care should be taken to avoid injury to the snake or handler.

If the snake's head needs to be restrained for a particular purpose, for example a health examination or venom collection:

- It can be restrained from behind with the thumb and third finger on either side, gripping the base of the skull and the index finger on top of the head (Figure 14.6).
- The fourth and fifth finger can be used to support the neck region and prevent any abnormal pressure being applied to the joint between the skull and the cervical vertebrae.
- Most snakes will resist this grip, probably because they feel threatened. Predators would naturally attack a snake's head first, to immobilize it as quickly as possible. Therefore, to keep stress to a minimum, it is best to only use this grip when necessary and for as short a time as possible

Snakes are generally capable of striking at speeds much faster than people are capable of reacting. Extreme care should be taken when attempting this grip to avoid being bitten:

- Some handlers will place a snake on a flat surface, for example a rubber mat, and use a snake hook to momentarily pin the snake to the mat, just behind the head, to give them enough time to restrain the head without being bitten.
- This is both stressful to the snake and a difficult technique to perform.
- Too little pressure allows the snake to move out from under the hook and strike, while too much pressure can cause severe injury to the cervical region.

An alternative method for examining the head of an aggressive or venomous species is to use a snake tube:

- These are short lengths of clear plastic tubing. The width of the tube must be only slightly larger than the width of the snake at the widest point.

- The snake is encouraged into the end of the tube. This is normally relatively easy to accomplish, as snakes will often enter the tube as part of normal exploration/hunting behaviour, or for safety.
- When the snake has passed a sufficient way into the tube, the handler can grip the snakes body and tube at the entry point to prevent the snake going any further.
- At this point the snake can be visually examined with relative safety.
- The disadvantage of using this method is it can be difficult to ascertain the correct size of tube required. Too small and snakes may not want to enter, or they become lodged in the tube if allowed to advance too far. Too large and they are able to turn around inside the tube and move back towards the handler.
- Tubes are not appropriate for some species, for example Boomslang or King Cobra (and other elapids), and a squeeze box may be necessary for handling in these cases (Fowler, 2008).

14.3 Restraint and Handling of Lizards

14.3.1 Anatomical Considerations

There is a wide variation in morphology between different species, ranging from those with specialized adaptations for hunting, such as chameleons, to legless lizards, such as the slow worm. This chapter focuses on handling small-to-medium-sized lizards commonly found in captivity. As previously mentioned, some species are venomous, so handlers should always identify species before attempting to restrain them. Many species also have defensive adaptations, such as modified scales, forming spikey protuberances around their head and body, as well as sharp claws on their feet.

14.3.2 Handling

Where individuals are not accustomed to being handled, alternatives to handling should always be considered in order to reduce the likelihood of causing stress or physical damage to the animal. Small lizards can be encouraged into clear containers, where they can easily be inspected or moved to another enclosure, without needing to be picked up. However, when handling is unavoidable, the time in hand should be kept to a minimum.

Always handle lizards over a table or close to the ground to prevent them from sustaining damage if they manage to escape the handler's grip.

As mentioned previously, lizards should never be handled by their tail due to the potential for autotomy to occur. However, large species, or those with long tails, should have the tail gently restrained under the handlers arm. This will reduce the likelihood of a tail becoming injured or being used to inflict injury on the handler.

Generally, the technique used for handling depends on the size of the lizard.

Medium sized lizards, such as Bearded Dragons, should be restrained with two hands (Figure 14.7). Similar to snakes, it is usually best to approach the lizard from behind to reduce the likelihood that it will feel threatened.

The handler's dominant hand is placed over the lizard's shoulders and the handler's fingers are used to gently restrain the forelegs so that they are brought backwards to lie against the body wall. The hand should be far enough forwards to prevent the lizard from

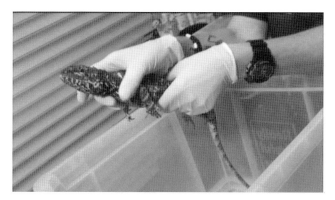

Figure 14.7 Restraint of a medium size lizard (Source: Courtesy of Marwell Zoo, 2016).

being able to turn and bite the handler. The other hand is placed over the lizard's lower back and pelvis and the fingers and thumb used to gently bring the hind leg backwards to lie alongside the tail.

Small lizards can be restrained using a one-handed modification of the technique described above. Similar to medium sized lizards, the handler approaches from behind the animal and uses the first finger and thumb to gently restrain across the shoulders. The rest of the lizards' body is gently cupped using the remaining fingers to hold the legs backwards against the body, but leaving the tail free. As small lizards can move extremely quickly, it is often advisable to hold them over a container in case they escape from the handler's grip.

14.4 Restraint and Handling of Chelonians

14.4.1 Anatomical Considerations

The spinal column and rib cage of tortoises and turtles have adapted to form a hard shell that provides protection for body organs. The top half of the shell is referred to as the carapace and the bottom half is called the plastron. Although the shell affords greater protection, its relative weight and inflexibility means that, unlike other reptiles, tortoises and turtles tend to be slower moving and do not climb well. The shell varies significantly between species depending on their specific adaptations. Some have soft shells or are unable to retract their head and legs fully while others may have hinge-like adaptation on the shell to reduce the opening once the head and legs are retracted. From a handler's perspective, the protection afforded by the carapace and plastron reduces the risk of damaging soft tissues through handling. However, handlers should be aware that the shell is composed of living tissue with a nerve supply that allows the tortoise or turtle to detect even a very light touch.

Chelonia have powerful musculature in their limbs relative to their size, which they use for activities such as digging or swimming. Large tortoises can retract their limbs very quickly and are capable of trapping fingers (or in the case of giant species, a whole hand). Most chelonia have claws that they can use very effectively to deter anyone who handles them. Some species, particularly turtles, may attempt to bite handlers.

14.4.2 Handling

Perhaps because this group of reptiles is relatively easier to handle than other groups, handlers can often make the mistake of not using the appropriate care or respect when handling. As with other species, tortoises and turtles would never normally be handled in the wild except when being predated, so handling may elicit a defensive behaviour, such as retracting into the shell, even in individuals handled regularly. In all cases, when handled, individuals should be kept horizontal and they should not ordinarily be turned or placed upside down.

- Medium sized chelonia should be handled with two hands at all times. Hands should generally be placed on either side, behind the front legs with fingers under the plastron and thumbs over the carapace (Figures 14.8 and 14.9).
- Individuals should always be kept close to the ground or a suitable surface in case they slip out of the handler's grasp (Figure 14.10).
- Very small chelonia can be picked up with one hand spanning the carapace using a thumb and one or two fingers on either side. The individual can then be placed on the palm of the other hand to provide support. This will also make them feel more secure.
- Large chelonia usually require several people for handling purposes. In some cases specialized lifting equipment may be necessary. Some species can inflict serious injury on handlers, for example snapping turtles. These require special handling techniques and should only be handled by experienced people (Fowler, 2008).
- Some long necked species of turtle are capable of reaching around to bite hands placed behind the front legs. In these species it may be possible to grip the carapace and plastron from behind the back legs on either side of the tail, although this technique should not be used if it compromises the grip of the handler or the support of the animal's weight.

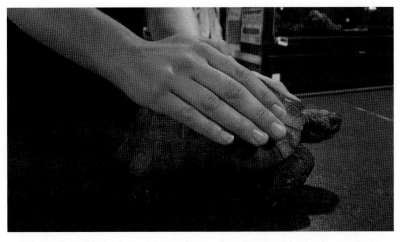

Figure 14.8 Handling a tortoise (Source: Courtesy of Brinsbury Campus, Chichester College).

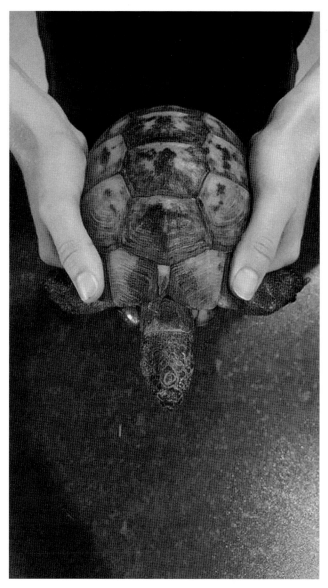

Figure 14.9 Handling a tortoise (Source: Courtesy of Brinsbury Campus, Chichester College).

Key Points

- Handling techniques vary considerably between different species of reptiles.
- It is reasonable to assume that handling may induce a stress response.
- Some lizards are capable of performing tail autotomy and should, therefore, not be handled by the tail.
- Venomous species should only be handled by experienced people, with assistance and the appropriate antivenin available in case of a bite injury.

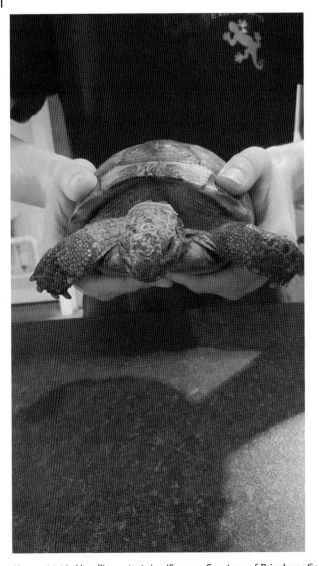

Figure 14.10 Handling a tortoise (Source: Courtesy of Brinsbury Campus, Chichester College).

- Large species of reptile can be dangerous due to their size and may require multiple people for handling. Some may also require special handling techniques not covered in this book. Always consider asking a more experience handler for advice before attempting to handle a species you are unfamiliar with.

Self-assessment Questions

1 What is the purpose of tail autotomy and why is it important to know whether a species is capable of performing it?

2   What should snakes be checked for prior to handling?

3   Describe a commonly used handling grip for medium sized tortoises?

4   Name three things a handler should have before attempting to handle a venomous snake?

Answers can be found in the back of the book.

References

BVA (2015) Policy statement on non-traditional companion animals. https://www.bva.co .uk/uploadedFiles/Content/News,_campaigns_and_policies/Policies/ Companion_animals/non-traditional-companion-animal-policy-position.pdf; last accessed 2 June 2017.

Fowler, M.E. (2008) *Restraint and Handling of Wild and Domestic Animals*, 3rd edn, John Wiley & Sons, Inc, Hoboken, NJ.

PFMA (2015) Pet Population Statistics 2014–15. Pet Food Manufacturers Association, London (http://www.pfma.org.uk/pet-population-2015; last accessed 2 June 2017).

Further Reading

Fowler, M.E. and Miller, R.E. (2003) *Zoo and Wild Animal Medicine*, 5th edn, Saunders.

Girline, S.J. (2013) *Veterinary Nursing of Exotic Pets*, 2nd edn, John Wiley & Sons Ltd, Chichester.

UK Government (1976) Dangerous Wild Animals Act 1976. http://www.legislation.gov.uk/ ukpga/1976/38; last accessed 2 june 2017.

Mader, D. (2006) *Reptile Medicine and Surgery*, 2nd edn, Saunders.

Glossary

Allomarking a behaviour pattern in which an animal applies some scent-marking substance to its own species.

Biocontainment the containment of pathological microorganisms within a well-defined, strictly controlled area (usually a laboratory).

Biosecurity preventative measures designed to reduce the risk of transmission of infectious diseases.

Brachycephalic refers to the shape of a skull that is shorter than typical for its species. It is perceived as a desirable trait in some domesticated dog and cat breeds, for example Pugs, and can be normal or abnormal in other animal species.

Bunny burrito a method of restraint for a rabbit that involves wrapping the rabbit in a towel.

Carpal joint a series of small bones and joints equivalent to the wrist in humans.

Carrier an animal that harbours and transmits the causative agent of an infectious disease systemically but is asymptomatic or immune to it themselves.

Cast an animal lying in such a position that it is unable to return to its feet without assistance.

Chiffney bit also known as an anti-rearing bit. An in-hand bit designed for horses that are difficult to lead.

Classical conditioning a learning process that occurs when two stimuli are repeatedly paired.

Companion animal term used to refer to any pet animal that is kept by humans for companionship and enjoyment.

Crepuscular active at dawn and dusk.

Cria name for a baby camelid.

Dichromate inability to see the colour red.

Disinfection clean with an agent in order to destroy bacteria.

Diurnal active both night and day.

Elbow the joint connecting the humerus, radius and ulna.

Feral an animal in a wild state, especially after escape from captivity or domestication.

Fomite objects or materials that are likely to carry infection, such as clothes, utensils and vehicles.

Habituation the diminishing of an innate response to a frequently repeated stimulus.

Hinny the offspring of a female donkey and a male horse.

Lagomorph a mammal of the order *Lagomorpha*, which comprises hares, rabbits and pikas.

Safe Handling and Restraint of Animals: A Comprehensive Guide, First Edition. Stella J. Chapman.
© 2018 John Wiley & Sons Ltd. Published 2018 by John Wiley & Sons Ltd.

Limbic system a complex system of nerves and networks in the brain involving several areas near the edge of the cortex concerned with instinct and mood. Controls the basic emotions of fear, pleasure and anger.

Neonatal term used to refer to new-born mammals.

Neophobic refers to the tendency of an animal to avoid or retreat from an unfamiliar object or situation.

Nocturnal active at night.

Obligate nasal breather an animal that breathes in and out via the nostrils only and not through the mouth, for example horse, cat and rabbit.

Operant conditioning a type of learning where behaviour is controlled by consequences.

Pathogen a bacteria, virus or other microorganism that can cause disease.

Pectoral muscle four large muscles found over the rib cage that play a primary role in flight in birds.

Pheromone a chemical substance produced and released into the environment by an animal that affects the behaviour or physiology of others of its species.

Progenitor an animal from which an animal is descended or originates; an ancestor or parent.

Pygostyle a bone formed from several fused tail vertebrae that support the tail feathers.

Recumbent refers to the position of an animal when lying down in a variety of positions, such as lateral (on the side) or sternal (on the sternum).

Sacrum a bone formed from several fused vertebrae connected to the pelvis.

Tail autotomy a process by which certain species of lizard will drop their tail if they feel threatened.

Temperament an animal's nature, especially as it permanently affects their behaviour.

Thermoregulation the process by which warm-blooded animals maintain their body temperature.

Tonic immobilization method of restraint occasionally used in rabbits; achieved by causing the rabbit to freeze and become unresponsive, which can cause stress.

Trachea the anatomical term for the windpipe.

Vector an organism, typically a biting insect or tick, that transmits a disease or parasite from one animal to another.

Zoonoses a disease that can be transmitted to humans from animals.

Answers to Chapter Questions

Chapter One: Biosecurity

1   What is a zoonotic disease?
    a *A disease transmitted from animals to humans.*

2   PPE is the abbreviation for?
    a *Personal Protective Equipment.*

3   What are the four basic principles to biosecurity?
    • *Selection of animals from known sources with known health status – of particular relevance to farm animals.*
    • *Isolation of new animals on arrival at the facility.*
    • *Movement control within the facility.*
    • *Sanitation using disinfection of materials and equipment and good personal hygiene.*

4   What are standard operating procedures (SOPs)?

    These are detailed written instructions that can be used to satisfy compliance requirements and are recommended for all procedures that pose a potential risk to the health and safety of personnel. They should also be used as the base for everyday training of staff.

5   Why is good hand hygiene important and when should you ensure that you wash your hands?

    Hands should be washed to prevent spread of disease between animals and to humans. Hot water and soap should be used and a good hand washing protocol, such as the World Health Organization (WHO) hand washing protocol, should ideally be followed. Hands should be washed at the following times:
    • *before and after handling animals and leaving the facility between different animals or species;*
    • *before and after toilet or lunch break periods;*
    • *after glove removal and handling chemicals.*
    NB: Hand gel or rub may be used, unless hands are visibly soiled.

Safe Handling and Restraint of Animals: A Comprehensive Guide, First Edition. Stella J. Chapman.
© 2018 John Wiley & Sons Ltd. Published 2018 by John Wiley & Sons Ltd.

Chapter Two: Welfare

1 What are the key differences between the five freedoms and five needs?

Whilst the five freedoms were developed initially to address the welfare of farm animals, the five needs of the Animal Welfare Act (2006) arose in order to consider the welfare of all animals and to impose a 'duty of care' to owners and those responsible for the care of animals. The 'five freedoms' were also developed as a measure of poor welfare, whereas the 'five needs' strive to highlight what an animal needs in order to demonstrate good welfare.

2 Give examples of species that are now referred to as non-traditional companion animals.

Birds, reptiles and small mammals, such as rodents.

3 Which physiological parameters can be looked at in animals to measure the stress response to handling?

Cortisol, glucose and lactate.

4 What is the function of the stria terminalis?

This is the part of the brain that is involved with the emotional response of separation distress.

Chapter Three: Dogs

1 What is meant by the term 'critical period'?

'Critical' period refers to the time when a small amount of experience (or a total lack of experience) will have an effect on later behaviour.

2 Why is the socialization period for puppies so important in terms of behaviour?

From a behavioural point of view, the socialization period is most important as it is during this time that puppies learn about their environment and about humans, with key behaviours being play (highest frequency during this time), dominance (with littermates), avoidance behaviour and, by eight weeks of age, fear reactions.

3 When approaching a dog, what general principles should be applied?
   - *The environment should be safe and secure.*
   - *The dog should be encouraged to approach the handler rather than the handler imposing themselves.*
   - *Direct eye contact should be avoided.*

- *Threatening postures such as leaning over or cornering should be avoided. Crouching down to the dog's level may be less intimidating but care should be taken to avoid the risk of facial injury to the handler.*
- *Calm and simple voice commands may reassure the dog and focus its attention.*
- *Treats may be given as distractors and rewards but should be offered with permission of the owner. The dog may have dietary sensitivities, or the owner may prefer that treats are not given.*

4   Name five pieces of equipment that might be used in a kennel environment to control a dog that is being handled or moved.

Slip lead, collar and lead, choke chain, halter, harness, muzzle, towel, dog catcher.

5   State 3 behaviours that an anxious but submissive dog might display.

Blinking/squinting, low tail carriage, shaking, panting, low ear carriage, slow tail wag, lip/nose licking, yawning, rolling onto back, averting eye contact, reluctance to play or take treats.

Chapter Four: Cats

1   What is meant by the term socialization and what age is regarded as the kittens 'sensitive' period for socialization?

Socialization is the term used to describe the process of development of potentially advantageous behavioural changes as a result of exposure to novel situations involving people, other animals and new environments. 2–7 weeks of age is regarded as the feline 'sensitive' period for socialization, which is earlier than that of dogs.

2   State three behaviours you might see in a relaxed cat.

Lying curled up or on side, tail loosely wrapped if lying and curled at tip if standing, eyes half closed, purring, ears relaxed, slow blink, pupils' small.

3   What additional items of equipment might you use to restrain a fractious or difficult cat?

Towel, cat net, cat bag, towel, cat muzzle, crush cage, pheromone diffuser, gauntlets, cat catcher.

4   State three things you would do before removing a cat from a cage.

Check the environment is secure – doors and windows closed; check no other animals loose or a potential risk; check personnel safe (children etc.); observe behaviour/health prior to handling.

5   House cats rub themselves against their owner's legs in order to?
   a *Scent mark*

Chapter Five: Rabbits

1   Which of these methods of restraint is most appropriate for general examination of a rabbit?
    a *Towel wrap*

2   Name two behaviours often shown by aggressive or stressed rabbits.

    Thumping of hind feet, grunting, growling, ears flat against head.

3   What anatomical considerations should be taken into account when handling rabbits?
    - *The rabbit's spine must always be supported in a normal position to maintain the normal curvature of the spine at all times to prevent vertebral factures.*
    - *The hind limbs must always be supported and controlled, as rabbits can cause serious injury and deep wounds to the handler if they kick.*
    - *Similarly, rabbits should be released from restraint slowly and only when all feet are on the ground, to prevent injury to the rabbit or handler by kicking.*

4   'Trancing' is a method that has been described for the restraint of rabbits. Under what circumstance might you consider this restraint method and why should it not be used as a general method for restraining rabbits?

    'Trancing' is sometimes advocated as a method of restraint of relaxation in rabbits. This is a fear response, which causes stress and is rarely necessary in rabbit handling. It can be achieved by placing a rabbit in dorsal recumbency and stroking the head. This will cause the rabbit to freeze and become unresponsive to stimuli. It should never be used to perform painful procedures but can be used as a last resort in aggressive or fearful rabbits.

Chapter Six: Rodents

1   Which of the following is NOT a normal guinea pig behaviour?
    d. *Thumping*

2   Which rodent species is NOT at risk to deglove the tail when handled?
    a *Hamster*

3   Define the terms (i) crepuscular, (ii) nocturnal and (iii) diurnal, and state which rodents belong in which category.

    Rodents can be crepuscular (active at dawn and dusk) i.e. hamsters; diurnal (active both day and night) i.e. gerbils; or nocturnal (active at night) i.e. rats and mice.

4   Discuss how rodents use smell to communicate.

Smell – rodents use scent marking in many social contexts including inter- and intraspecies communication, in order to mark trails and establish territories. The odour of a predator will depress this behaviour. They are able to recognize close relatives and this allows them to show preferential behaviour (nepotism) toward their kin and also to avoid in-breeding. Hamsters, in particular, become very accustomed to the scent of the group, and if one hamster is extensively handled the group may attack it.

5   For which species of rodent may scruffing be considered necessary and why?

Scruffing may be necessary for aggressive hamsters. The handler's thumb and forefingers grasp the loose skin over the shoulders, whilst the remaining fingers support the hamsters' bodyweight and the other hand supports the hindquarters.

Chapter Seven: Ferrets

1   Discuss the ways in which ferrets communicate.
- *Vocalization – ferrets produce a variety of different noises, that is hiss and chuckle (playing), scream (fighting, frightened or threatened) and grumble (foraging).*
- *Vision – ferrets have relatively poor vision and, as a consequence of this, their natural instinct is to nip at objects that move in their field of vision. This is important for handlers to be aware of, as they may bite if they do not see what is in front of them.*
- *Scent – ferrets are carnivores and use smell to hunt. They also use scent to communicate with each other.*

2   Why is it important the ferrets are socialized from an early age?

In the wild ferrets spend a large proportion of their time foraging and have wide home ranges, thus ferrets are naturally very active. They are intelligent and thus need mental as well as physical stimulation; this is very important in young ferrets, as play is required for them to develop motor and social skills, in addition to learning and predatory behaviours. Good socialization is very important for ferrets in order to prepare them for life in a human environment. Handlers need to understand that ferrets:
- *are highly motivated and need to explore and forage;*
- *require adequate resting opportunities and play opportunities;*
- *social organization of groups is important in order to decrease interspecies and territorial aggression.*

3   Describe how you would handle a ferret on a table for examination.

Put the ferret on a table with the handler's index and middle fingers placed over the ferret's shoulders and the handler's remaining fingers restraining the ferret's body.

The handler's thumb should be behind the ferret's elbow to prevent the ferret from moving backwards. The handler's other hand should be placed over the hindquarters to provide extra restraint

4 Describe how you would restrain an aggressive ferret.

Aggressive ferrets may be handled with gauntlets to prevent injury to the handler. Ferrets may also be scruffed if necessary. Many procedures can be performed by distracting the ferret with high quality cat food, fed on a tongue depressor. This will enable the handler to perform tasks such as nail clips and physical examination.

Chapter Eight: Horses

1 How is handling of the donkey influenced by the fact that naturally they can live solitary lives?

Living solitary lives means that it is ineffective for a donkey to run away from a predator, so they will stand still and observe the situation. This time of observing allows them to work out what the best response to the situation is. With regards to handling, this principle must also be applied. When the donkey is unsure of the situation, it will stand its ground. A donkey must be given time to assess any task that is being asked of it to ensure its welfare is maintained.

2 With regards to handling, what is the importance of the bond between a pair of donkeys?

Donkeys have very strong social bonds and should be kept together at all times where possible. Donkeys that are separated from their companions can become stressed very easily and this can make handling difficult. In addition, a donkey can become unwell when it is separated for a length of time from its companion due to the stress experienced.

3 How does placing a hand under the chin of the donkey prevent it from moving forward?

Placing a hand under the chin of the donkey allows the handler to have extra control, as donkeys follow the principal of where the head is, the body goes. The slight lifting of the head from the chin will prevent the donkey from going forward because its head is not in the forward position.

4 What are the dangers involved in holding a donkeys front leg for restraint?

The donkey is very agile and even when holding up a leg, a donkey can well place a kick, even when standing on two legs.

5   Why should the twitch only be used for short procedures and where (anatomically) is it recommended not to twitch a horse?

The use of the twitch has received attention in recent years due to its potential to be misused, despite it being a method of restraint that is commonly used in equine yards. The principle behind the use of the twitch is that it applies pressure to an area of the horse's skin that, as previously mentioned, has sensory nerves and acts by releasing endorphins from the central nervous system, thereby causing the horse to relax. The twitch should only be used for short procedures. The controversy around the use of the twitch is with regards to the fact that when applied to certain areas of the horses' body, that is ear and upper lip, a degree of pain is to be expected and it is the pain of application that horses are responding to. When used incorrectly, the twitch can also be associated with learned and aversive behaviours, that is the horse becomes head-shy following the application of an ear twitch. It is recommended that ear twitching is not done on any horse or donkey.

6   How would you restrain a foal?

When restraining a foal it is important not to place too much pressure on the head, as this can often lead to frustration and aversive behaviour by the foal. It is much better to simply encircle the foal with one arm placed around the chest and the other around behind the hindquarters. With an older or bigger foal, placing the foal against a wall and putting a knee firmly into the flank is usually enough to keep it still. It is important to be quiet and calm with foals, as they can move very quickly and will buck and rear in order to try to escape the handler. Also, be very mindful of the mare, as if mare feels that its foal is being threatened it will become anxious and may even be aggressive towards the handler.

Chapter Nine: Cattle

1   What is the flight zone?

The flight zone is an area around the cow that dictates that cows' personal space. When it is entered by a handler, the cow will move away from the handler in order to maintain that personal space.

2   Describe what optimal pressure means.

Optimal pressure is the amount of pressure required to move an animal in any direction at its own pace.

3   Describe how to restrain a calf.

A calf can be restrained in a number of ways. If it is halter trained, it may be that this is the only amount of restraint required. If the calf is not haltered trained and is small enough, it can be held by placing one arm around the front chest and neck area and the other around the back end by the tail. If further restraint is required, a calf can be placed onto its side and its front and back feet tied together to prevent it from standing. If an assistant is available, the calf can be simply held on its side by placing a knee over the shoulder and holding down the top front and back legs.

4   Why use curved chutes?

Curved chutes use the principle of following the leader. The lead cow moves into the curved chute and the others follow behind to the point that the lead cow can no longer turn back around. Cattle move in a circular motion so that they return to where they were previously and this is the principle used for the design of a curved chute.

5   Where is the point of balance?

The point of balance on an individual cow is at the shoulder. A point of balance for a herd of cattle is the point at which the group will turn when pressure is applied.

Chapter Ten: Small Ruminants

1   Describe the process you would use to move a group of sheep.

Always try to keep a group of sheep together. Take advantage of their flocking instinct by giving them time to keep together. Dogs, vehicles or handlers should work in a semicircular motion behind the sheep, stepping into their flight zone and keeping behind the point of balance (shoulder) to keep them going forward and using this area to move the flock left or right as needed. Slow, deliberate movements will keep the sheep calm and will make them easier to move.

2   Rather than 'cut' an individual or small group from the rest of the flock, what is a better way to separate an individual for examination?

Rather than cutting an individual or small group from the rest of the flock using a dog, it is better to move the entire group through a race and use a special sorting gate. This will reduce the stress overall.

3   What are the key considerations when gathering sheep off a hill?

Sheep that are gathered from the hill are likely to have not been handled often, so will experience high stress levels. It is important that any gather is well planned and that the sheep are allowed to go at their own pace. This especially applies when there are lambs at foot as they can tire very easily. Keep the sheep moving at a steady pace and rest when required. Note must be taken of the weather conditions and terrain.

4 What is the difference between sheep and goats in terms of flocking instinct and how does this affect the way a group is moved?

Sheep have a very strong flocking instinct and will want to stay together. They can be driven as a group from behind. Goats, on the other hand, although they do having a grouping instinct, do not have as strong a flocking instinct. Goats cannot be moved from behind and should be moved from the front, either through the use of lead goat or through encouragement with food to come forward towards the handler.

5 Goats should never be placed on their rumps. Explain why.

Goats should never be placed on their rumps because they do not have the same fat coverage as sheep, so it can cause injury and bruising.

6 Name three similar ways you can restrain a goat or sheep.

Both goats and sheep can be restrained in the following manner:
i) *One hand under the chin or around the chest, the other hand around the rump/tail.*
ii) *Against a wall with one hand under the chin and the other hand placed on the rump with one leg placed against the flank. The other leg can be placed at shoulder for extra restraint.*
iii) *Both a well-trained goat and sheep can be restrained with the use of a head collar.*

Chapter Eleven: Pigs

1 Why are pigs prone to overheating?

Pigs cannot sweat, so this is why they are prone to overheating.

2 How do you build trust with a pig?

Placing a firm and gentling hand on the back of pig regularly can help to build trust. Calm and considerate handling goes a long way when working with pigs.

3 What is the best way to catch a piglet?

Piglets can be caught by carefully grasping at a back leg and then very quickly moving a hand to around the chest area and the other hand under the flank area. Then the piglet can be lifted up to the handlers' chest, where the hand under the flank reaches around and is placed upon the back of the piglet; the hand at the front is used to push the piglet gently into the chest of the handler. This will make it feel safe and secure.

4 How should a group of pigs be moved?

Pigs should be moved in small groups of three or four. The area in which the pigs are to be moved should be free from obstruction and the path should be clear ahead with non-slip floors. A small group of pigs can be moved through the use of a board, flags or rattles at the back of the group and pressure applied only when required. Simply walking calmly behind the animal entering the edge of its flight zone should keep a small group moving forwards without the need for extra force.

Chapter Twelve: Camelids

1 What is the primary defence reaction of a camelid and what methods can be used to avoid this?

The primary defence of a camelid is to regurgitate its stomach contents and spit towards the handler. Methods that can be used to avoid this are calm and confident handling, standing out of the way when there are behavioural signs that the animal is about to spit, cover the animals nose with a light weight cloth or towel (use with caution!).

2 What are 'extension wands' used for?

Extension wands are used to help guide a group or individual into a space. The wands are extensions to the handlers' arms. They should never be waved around or used to hit the animal.

3 Describe the key features of a good handling chute.

A good handling chute should be specially designed for the animal and the correct size for either a llama or an alpaca. Shoulder bars and a moveable back bar are key features of a good chute. It should be high enough to discourage jumping out of the area.

4 Outline the importance of a correctly fitting head collar.

The head collar must be fitted correctly on a llama or alpaca as they are semi-obligate nasal breathers, meaning that they can only breathe through their noses. Also, they do not have a protective bony part over their nasal cavities, so if the nose band is too low down on the nose it will restrict their breathing.

5 What is kushing and what are the welfare concerns associated with this?

Kushing means to sit down. Camelids that sit down on their own accord are highly likely to be stressed and any procedure should be carried out as quickly as possible before the animal is left alone to recover. If the animal needs to be restrained by kushing, this needs to be carried out in a very considerate and careful manner. The same principles should be applied above in that this position is likely to be highly stressful, so any procedure requiring this form of restraint should be carried out quickly and effectively.

Chapter Thirteen: Birds

1 Why is it important to draw curtains or pull blinds in the room before handling birds?

This is primarily to block out light from the windows, which helps to quieten the bird down and reduces stress. It also ensures that a bird will not try and fly towards a closed window should it get free of the handler's grip.

2 Why is it important to not hold birds too tightly around the body?

Birds have air sacs throughout their body that drive air back and forth through a rigid lung. These are easily compressed if handled too tightly, preventing the bird from breathing.

3 Why should birds be visually assessed prior to handling?

As birds are often very susceptible to the stress of handling, it is important to gauge the state the individual is in before attempting to handle it. Those showing high levels of stress should be allowed to calm down for a period of 30–60 minutes or longer before being handled. Any bird showing signs of illness should not be handled and veterinary attention should be sought.

4 Describe a grip commonly used to restrain passerines.

A 'three-fingered grip' can be used. The head is restrained between the first and second fingers while the thumb is brought around the front of the bird to hold it gently against the palm of the hand.

Chapter Fourteen: Reptiles

1 What is the purpose of tail autotomy and why is it important to know whether a species is capable of performing it?

This is a defensive behaviour shown by some species of lizard. The tail can be rapidly 'dropped' if grabbed by a predator. It will continue to move for a short time after being dropped to distract the predator, whilst the lizard runs away. Handlers should be aware of species that perform this behaviour, as they may accidently cause tail drop to occur. In these cases, the tail may grow back but will not look the same as previously.

2 What should snakes be checked for prior to handling?

Snakes should be assessed for any signs of abnormal behaviours or signs of aggression. They should also be checked to ensure that they are not going into shed and that they have not eaten recently.

3   Describe a commonly used handling grip for medium sized tortoises.

Hands are placed on either side of the shell behind the front legs, with thumbs on top of the carapace. Tortoises should be held in a horizontal position unless absolutely necessary. Keep them close to the floor, or another surface, in case they manage to escape the handler's grip.

4   Name three things a handler should have before attempting to handle a venomous snake?

Handlers must have broad experience of snake handling before attempting to handle venomous species. Antivenin, appropriate for the species, should be available at all times. An emergency bite protocol should be written and in place.

Index

Safe Handling and Restraint of Animals: A Comprehensive Guide, First Edition. Stella J. Chapman.
© 2018 John Wiley & Sons Ltd. Published 2018 by John Wiley & Sons Ltd.